Safe & Secure
SCHOOLS

Safe & Secure
SCHOOLS

27 Strategies for Prevention and Intervention

Judy M. Brunner
Dennis K. Lewis

A Joint Publication

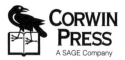

CORWIN PRESS
A SAGE Company

AMERICAN ASSOCIATION
OF SCHOOL ADMINISTRATORS

For information:

Corwin Press
A SAGE Company
2455 Teller Road
Thousand Oaks, California 91320
www.corwinpress.com

SAGE Ltd.
1 Oliver's Yard
55 City Road
London EC1Y 1SP
United Kingdom

SAGE India Pvt. Ltd.
B 1/I 1 Mohan Cooperative Industrial Area
Mathura Road, New Delhi 110 044
India

SAGE Asia-Pacific Pte. Ltd.
33 Pekin Street #02–01
Far East Square
Singapore 048763

Printed in the United States of America.

Library of Congress Cataloging-in-Publication Data

Brunner, Judy M.
Safe & secure schools : 27 strategies for prevention and intervention/Judy M. Brunner, Dennis K. Lewis.
    p. cm.
"A joint publication with the American Association of School Administrators (AASA)."
Includes bibliographical references and index.
ISBN 978-1-4129-6298-8 (cloth)
ISBN 978-1-4129-6299-5 (pbk.)
    1. Schools—Safety measures—Handbooks, manuals, etc. 2. Schools—Security measures—Handbooks, manuals, etc. I. Lewis, Dennis K. II. Title.

LB2864.5.B78 2009
363.11'9371—dc22   2008017909

This book is printed on acid-free paper.

            14   10   9   8   7   6   5   4   3

Acquisitions Editor:	Hudson Perigo
Editorial Assistant:	Lesley K. Blake
Production Editor:	Libby Larson
Copy Editor:	Alison Hope
Typesetter:	C&M Digitals (P) Ltd.
Proofreader:	Dorothy Hoffman
Indexer:	Sylvia Coates
Cover Designer:	Lisa Miller
Graphic Designer:	Karine Hovsepian

Contents

Foreword

Nothing makes headlines more quickly than a school shooting. Such an event violates an iconic safe haven and prompts parents in every community to wonder, "Could it happen here?" Suddenly popular media outlets are activated, archived Columbine footage is flashed across TV screens, and school safety consultants are answering insistent questions: "Are schools safe? Are we investing enough in security personnel and equipment? Or—gasp—do we need a national policy?"

"These kinds of situations are just like terrorist situations," National Association of Secondary School Principals (NASSP) Specialist for School Safety Bill Bond said on the occasion of one school shooting. "When people have so much hate in them that they don't mind dying, you don't have any deterrents left. People want to have metal detectors and security guards and all of this, but the real thing that makes a difference is working with the kids and adjusting to the kids" (personal communication, October 12, 2005).

Bond's comments strike a stark contrast between how school safety is considered by the general public and by school leaders. For school leaders, safety isn't just about preventing a tragic event: It's about maintaining a personalized environment in which every student is known and feels valued. It's about providing opportunities for every student to be successful. It's about modeling and fostering a pervasive attitude—on the part of every adult and student in the school—that threatening and belittling behaviors have no place in any school.

Not surprisingly, the conditions that mitigate school violence are the same conditions that promote high academic achievement. *Breaking Ranks II* and *Breaking Ranks in the Middle* (NASSP 2004, 2006), NASSP's handbooks on reform in high schools and middle schools, respectively, call for a school culture centered around personalization because, to quote educational reformer Ted Sizer (1999), "We cannot teach students well if we do not know them well" (p. 6). And knowing every student well encourages educators to work through their frustrations so that, even if those frustrations have not been resolved, at least they have been aired constructively.

From 2004 to 2007, members of the NASSP were regularly reminded of these themes in the "Safety Tips for Principals" column in *Principal Leadership* magazine. To their credit, column authors Dennis Lewis and Judy Brunner address the spectrum of safety issues—from the day-to-day behaviors that foster a positive climate, to warning signs of violence, to the specifics of crisis preparedness and response.

I commend Dennis and Judy on their work to ensure safe environments in schools and further commend them for taking their guidance to a broader audience. While the principal can provide leadership, it is only with a cooperative effort on the part of all with a stake in school success that educators can create truly personalized environments and can anticipate a day when news of a school shooting no longer hits the headlines.

Dr. Gerald Tirozzi, Executive Director
National Association of Secondary School Principals

Acknowledgments

Since the conception in 1999 of Edu-Safe LLC, a school safety consulting firm, several individuals and organizations have made significant contributions to the growth of our business, as well as to our own professional development. We are very grateful to them for allowing us the opportunity to submit articles for publication, present papers at conferences, and provide staff development to education professionals across the United States.

Three individuals that have been especially helpful are Jan Umphrey, editor of NASSP's *Principal Leadership*; Jim King, executive director of Missouri Association of Secondary School Principals; and Elizabeth Brenkus, former acquisitions editor for Corwin Press. Jan was the first to give us a national forum for our ideas and suggestions related to school safety and security through the column "Safety Tips for Principals." Jim was always willing to provide ideas and suggestions for statewide professional opportunities, and Lizzie was never too busy to provide guidance and encouragement at times when we needed it most. We are very grateful for her professional demeanor, smiling face, and positive attitude.

We are also grateful to the following professional organizations:

National Association of Secondary School Principals

National Association of School Safety and Law Enforcement Officers

American Association of School Administrators

Missouri Association of Secondary School Principals

Springfield Missouri Public Schools

Last, but not least, we wish to thank our families and friends for being patient when our professional obligations and responsibilities took time, effort, and perseverance.

About the Authors

Judy M. Brunner and **Dennis K. Lewis** are authors and consultants on a variety of topics related to school safety and security. They are cofounders of Edu-Safe LLC (www.edu-safe.org), a school safety and advisory organization providing professional development and resources to school personnel across the United States.

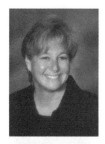 **Ms. Brunner** is a former high school, middle school, and elementary school principal, and is currently an adjunct instructor at Missouri State University. She is a nationally recognized authority and speaker on the topics of school safety and security, and prevention of bullying behaviors. She provides technical and training assistance for a number of state and national organizations.

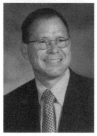 **Mr. Lewis** is the past president and chairman of the Board of the National Association of School Safety and Law Enforcement Officers, and is a nationally recognized authority and speaker on the topics of school safety, site risk assessments, and bullying prevention. He is the former director of school police for the Springfield, Missouri Public Schools and provides technical and training assistance for a number of state and national organizations.

Judy Brunner and Dennis Lewis can be reached at edusafe@edu-safe.org.

Introduction

Schools of the twenty-first century are expected to provide a level of security unprecedented in the history of education. With a backdrop of increasingly prevalent violent behavior in society that has spilled over into schools, there is often a clash between the need to secure campuses and the desire to maintain an open and welcoming environment. As schools have responded with a myriad of strategies designed to strengthen security in and around campuses, some individuals call for more drastic measures, claiming not enough is being done, while others say schools have already gone too far.

While academic achievement should always be the primary focus of all who work in the school, great school leaders recognize that for this to be accomplished, a number of support columns must be in place. School safety is one of the columns supporting this mission; its removal or damage can have negative and even devastating consequences on academic achievement.

Although acts of school violence resulting in loss of life are still rare, students, staff, and parents are well aware of the headlines. These headlines can erode the confidence of parents hundreds of miles away from a specific event. In the aftermath of any school tragedy, school personnel self-evaluate and consider whether or not they have done enough to prevent such an occurrence on their own campus.

Safe school planning must merge two important concepts if it is to truly make a difference. First, a physical environment must be created that is reasonably safe. Second, the environment must be perceived as safe by the entire school community. Both concepts are challenging but equally important. Planning should not only address concrete items such as locks, doors, windows, parking lots, and lighting, but should also include strategies on how to promote these to the school community, while giving everyone ownership in the process.

THE GOAL OF THIS BOOK

The strategies in this book were originally written as columns for the NASSP's *Principal Leadership*. They have been edited to appeal to a wider audience, as well as to reflect the most up-to-date best practices. It is our intent to provide you, the reader, with the knowledge and tools to create and enhance a safe learning environment for students, staff, and the patrons who periodically visit your campus. We have attempted to do so by

- providing tips and strategies that have minimal or no associated cost;
- using strategies that blend with the educational atmosphere of most schools and are acceptable to most school communities;
- structuring the suggestions so implementation can be accomplished without major time commitments, while keeping the focus on academic achievement; and
- recommending methods of enhancing school safety we believe can make a difference in preventing or minimizing the opportunity for a tragedy to occur, facilitating a better response should such an event happen, and allowing a school to recover and return to normalcy in the aftermath of such an event.

Safe & Secure Schools: 27 Strategies for Prevention and Intervention provides a foundation for safe school planning. While not intended to address every security issue or problem faced by schools in the twenty-first century, the strategies provided in this book, when incorporated with systematic planning, ongoing discussion, and a review process, can make a positive difference.

WHO THIS BOOK IS FOR

While the primary audience for this book is the school administrator, there are a number of other individuals that can benefit from the content. In fact, following the concept promoted by the authors that it is critical to make everyone in a school building "participatory to the process," all staff members should read it. There are some groups and individuals that should be targeted specifically: Safety coordinators or individuals who, by job classification, have a specific responsibility for developing, planning, and implementing safe school strategies will find the book a valuable resource. Staff contemplating a future career move into administration will find the contents thought provoking. And, for schools that use safety committees, ad hoc groups, or other teams of individuals (such as counselors, school social workers, and lead teachers) to help guide safe school planning, the strategies and concepts contained in the following chapters will provide a starting point for discussion toward mapping out a course of action. Regardless of the audience, there is something for everyone with a vested interest in enhancing school safety.

WHAT THIS BOOK IS NOT

Without belaboring the point, this book is not a cure or magic pill that will somehow fix or prevent the negative events that occasionally happen at school. Utilizing some or all of the strategies contained within is much like taking a daily aspirin to help prevent a heart attack. Bad events may still occur, but great leaders using the right medicine and following the prescription label help to minimize the opportunity.

HOW THIS BOOK IS ORGANIZED

The book is divided into four sections—planning, response strategies, professional development, and our recommended top ten strategies. While each chapter is related to these broad topics, some sections could easily be placed into more than one category. It was our intent to offer practical and cost-effective suggestions that principals could read "on the run." It is our hope this goal has been accomplished.

The final section of the book is titled, "Top Ten School Safety Strategies." Of all the ideas suggested within this text, we consider these to be the most important.

1

Planning

STRATEGY 1

Starting the School Year

A Checklist for Safety and Security

Creating a checklist before the school year begins helps ensure school safety procedures are in place and implemented throughout the school year.

As schools across the country prepare for the start of school each September, school officials know safety and security issues related to public and private education continue to change and evolve. Local and international events have put school personnel in the position of needing to continually emphasize and reassure students, staff, and their communities that school still provides an environment of normalcy and routine in the lives of all. In fact, school may be the only predictable environment for some students. School superintendents, principals, and teachers must go the extra mile to ensure that every reasonable and prudent precaution is taken to make certain the school is always a safe place for students.

FOLLOWING A SAFETY CHECKLIST

One of the ways administrators can accomplish this important mission is to create a checklist of safety tasks before the school year begins. Just as a pilot checks a preflight list before rolling down the runway, it is important for school leaders to make changes before "taking off" into the new school year. Once "in flight," it may be more difficult to make a correction.

Suggested checklist tasks include the following:

• Review the school's crisis management plan. This should include a start-up meeting with the emergency response team before the school year begins. Do not forget to include staff who are listed as alternates in the plan. Alternates should be just as familiar with the plan and specific responsibilities as are their designated counterparts.

• Use tabletop exercises for staff development. Because it is important for the entire emergency response team to engage in problem solving for specific security and safety-related scenarios as part of the practice and planning process, the emergency response team should take part in tabletop exercises at the start of the school year.

• Meet with representatives of local law enforcement agencies to discuss school safety issues. These meetings provide a good opportunity to exchange information on safety issues that may directly or indirectly affect the school community. Be sure to provide law enforcement representatives with a list of all anticipated major school activities for the coming school year. Send them updates during the year, as necessary. Many law enforcement agencies will give this information to area patrol officers so that added attention can be given to those school events.

• Communicate with community agencies that have a vested interest in the school's safety. These groups include juvenile authorities, health department agencies, and the local fire department. The purpose of this dialogue is to review any interagency agreements, new rules, or laws that pertain to the school. This is also a good opportunity to update contact information and to meet new staff members in those agencies. These contacts can be invaluable throughout the school year.

• Review existing laws and inform the administrative team and staff members of any new laws, court decisions, district policies, or practices that affect school safety and discipline. It is important to dedicate a portion of the first faculty meeting for reviewing this information. Do not forget to keep documentation about these meetings. In the aftermath of a critical incident, this information could be vital to everyone involved.

• Review the school's access-control measures, including the check-in procedures for visitors. Make certain appropriate signage is in place. If changes need to be made in procedures, it is generally less problematic for the public if they are made during the summer and implemented before the start of a new school year.

• Review all safety-related work orders. It is important for the principal or his designee to review all safety-related work orders prior to the first day of school. If critical repairs have not been completed, the principal should make appropriate contacts related to completion date and any interim measures necessary to ensure safety.

• Audit all first aid supplies and crisis management kits within the school to verify they are properly stocked and in their designated locations. Perishable items, such as batteries for flashlights and radios, should be replaced or recharged. Verify that the location of each kit is identified in the school's floor plan.

• Ensure that the school's floor plan includes any recent building modifications, including the plans previously supplied to emergency service providers. This will assist those agencies if they need to respond to the school during a critical incident.

• Verify that each classroom has all emergency information in place or posted, to include fire evacuation routes, sheltering locations, and emergency flip charts. This information should also be provided to each substitute teacher during the school year. To facilitate this process, a classroom check-list (see Resources) can be created so that each staff member can audit the classroom environment for the necessary items. Having faculty members participate in this process will add to their sense of ownership of the school's safety program.

• New staff members should receive in-service training on the various safety components and strategies of the school, and returning staff members should be reminded of these strategies. Do not overlook basic training, such as how to use a fire extinguisher, first aid procedures, and the class-room emergency-response flip chart.

• Review and analyze last year's discipline statistics and campus crime incidents. Review the statistics for possible trends involving specific infractions and the locations where they occurred. Review student and staff accident reports to determine if there is any causation commonality.

• Remind teachers to discuss appropriate safety procedures and security measures with their students. This discussion should occur during the first week of school as a part of the teacher's classroom orientation. Teachers should thoroughly review with all students their responsibilities related to reporting incidents of school violence. This can include hotline numbers and other anonymous reporting methods available to them.

• The principal should discuss and explain security and safety measures in use at the school during school orientations for students, parents, or guardians. This information should also be included in the student handbook, teacher handbook, and school website as part of the school's safety portfolio. This strategy can provide reassurance to all that school safety is a priority.

Although the summer months provide time for school administrators to reflect and review the past year's accomplishments, reflection alone is not enough. School leaders should strategically plan safety procedures as part of their overall decision-making process. A safety checklist provides an excellent method to ensure a quality-controlled beginning to each school year.

STRATEGY 2

The Principal's Homework

*What Does Your Teacher Handbook Say
About Safety and Security?*

Ensure that your teacher handbook addresses safety and security concerns. Schools now almost always provide a written handbook for teachers and certificated staff members. Administrators should make certain the handbook is reviewed and updated at least once each year. The most important aspect of the handbook, however, is that all teachers have a copy of the most up-to-date edition, that they have signed for receipt of it, and that they are held accountable for the information within. Copies also should be distributed to substitute teachers, student teachers, and teacher aides.

Because the teacher handbook is one of the primary methods of communicating administrative expectations, it provides the perfect opportunity to outline important safety and security information. The following checklist is not inclusive, but it does include what we consider minimal information related to safety and security. Use it to review your current teacher handbook.

• Administrative duties and responsibilities. The duties and responsibilities related to discipline and other assignments for each site administrator should be explained. If there is more than one site administrator, staff members need to understand which administrator oversees which specific tasks.

• Campus security expectations. If applicable, the handbook should explain how staff can enter and exit the building or campus after regular business hours. Information about working on the campus on weekends or holidays should be provided. The handbook is a good place to include information about access control for school classrooms, buildings, and campus during the school day.

• Key control. Schools should have a method of controlling and accounting for all keys that are issued to staff; all keys should be inventoried at least once a year. The handbook should include instructions for issuing keys, and what to do if building or classroom keys are lost or stolen during the school year.

• Procedures for reporting student attendance. This section should contain detailed procedures for reporting attendance. Definitions of and the appropriate faculty response for truancy and tardiness should be explained.

• Identification badges. The teacher handbook should explain the rules and regulations for displaying visual identification. If students are required to display or carry a picture badge, procedures for monitoring this practice should be in the handbook. If staff members must wear a picture badge or other identification, this requirement should also be included in the handbook.

• Disciplinary referrals and office procedures. Written guidelines for referring students to the office should be in the teacher handbook. Teachers should be encouraged to avoid using terms such as "defiant" and "disrespectful" in written referrals. For consistency and fairness, the teacher should refrain from prejudging the incident. Instead, the administrator should be the one to categorize the offense on the basis of the specific behavior described. Guidelines for contacting parents in a timely manner should also be given in the handbook.

• Visitor check-in procedures. Procedures for campus visitors should be detailed. Teachers should be directed to help maintain a closed campus by identifying and monitoring individuals who have not followed the appropriate protocol. Instructions for staff members on how to approach visitors when they observe them on campus should be in the handbook.

• Teacher check-in procedures; procedures for reporting teacher absence. Staff member check-in and check-out procedures should be in the handbook, along with a brief explanation of why these procedures are important. These should include time lines for how teachers should report a personal absence.

• Supervisory expectations. Included in the handbook should be detailed guidelines for teachers on supervising classrooms, hallways, the cafeteria, and restrooms. Instructions should include guidelines for teachers on supervision during assemblies and other activities. This section should also cover student passes, and whether and under what circumstances students are allowed to be in the hallways or common areas during class time.

• Guest speakers. If teachers are allowed to schedule classroom guest speakers, include in the teacher handbook guidelines for gaining administrative approval, along with check-in procedures for the guests.

• Student permission to leave campus. Write down the conditions under which students may leave the building or campus during the school day. High school handbooks should also contain procedures for going to the parking lot during the day.

• School nurse. How and under what conditions students are permitted to go to the school nurse should be outlined in the teacher handbook. If the nurse has specific office hours, they should be included in the handbook. This section should also contain regulations for dispensing student medication. All staff members should have a thorough understanding of acceptable and unacceptable possession and use of prescription and nonprescription drugs by students while on campus or at a school event.

• Lunch procedures. The handbook should address the lunch schedule, lunchroom procedures, and guidelines for supervising students during lunch.

• Assembly procedures. The handbook should provide procedures for attendance, entrance and exit, and behavior during assemblies. It should also state whether and under what circumstances staff is expected to attend assemblies, and their supervisory responsibilities.

• Field trips and cocurricular activities. Procedures for taking students off campus for a school activity—whether it is for an overnight or for a shorter trip during the school day—should be in the handbook. The handbook should also state that the following information is needed before the departure of any field trip:

   a. The name, address, and phone numbers of each student
   b. A printed itinerary of the trip
   c. Written permission from parents
   d. The trip time line
   e. Emergency medical forms
   f. The names of the chaperones, and copies of their security or background checks, as applicable
   g. Sponsor and chaperone expectations
   h. Transportation details
   i. Administrative approval

• Cash on campus. Teachers should be directed to never leave money in the classroom overnight. The handbook should outline how to deposit money collected for school activities, whether the deposit is made to a building financial secretary or a banking institution. Information about student fundraising can be included in this section.

• Instructions for substitute teachers. Teachers should be instructed to provide to the school office a folder containing instructions for substitute teachers. Each folder should include class seating charts, attendance procedures, disciplinary procedures, campus-level emergency plans, evacuation and sheltering procedures, safety and security information, and forms for disciplinary referrals.

- Parent and student handbook. Because teachers are often in a position of enforcing and explaining school rules to students during the school year, copies of parent and student handbooks should be issued to teachers along with the teacher handbook. Teachers should review the student handbook with their classes at the beginning of each year.

- Equipment inventory. The handbook should address the care, storage, and inventory of equipment. In particular, teachers should be directed to secure electronic devices when they are not in use. This section should also outline the storage of equipment during the summer months.

- Staff parking. If the school provides designated parking for staff members, the guidelines for parking should be in writing. This section should include information about parking permits, restricted areas, and other parking-related concerns.

After reviewing your handbook and comparing it to the checklist, how did you do? Did you "ace the test," or do you need to do some more handbook homework?

Everyone in school has homework from time to time, and school leaders are no exception. Those who procrastinate and fail to complete all the assignments could receive more than just a bad grade: they could find themselves in a potentially embarrassing position or, worse yet, in a situation that compromises student or staff safety. It is important that personnel review and revise the teacher handbook annually. This document will provide a written record of the expectations for staff and faculty.

STRATEGY 3

Strategic Supervision

The Foundation for School Safety

Well-planned supervision of students is the key to keeping them safe and preventing inappropriate behavior. Supervision is one of the basic building blocks of a safe and orderly school environment. Because supervision is such an essential component of a school safety program, it often becomes the focal point when something unfortunate happens, such as when a student is injured. Whether an injury occurs as a result of an accident or as the outcome of a confrontation with other students, the question of whether supervision was adequate may be asked.

The value of supervision is immeasurable in terms of monitoring and controlling student and adult behavior. Therefore, it is essential for school administrators to use every tool at their disposal to ensure the staff is properly educated and trained in how to supervise the students, and that the campus environment supports those efforts. Effective supervision begins with the guidance provided to staff members.

• Review the teacher handbook. The expectations for all staff who supervise students, including personnel in support roles, should be included in the teacher handbook.

• Staff should be present, alert, and in the hallways during class changes. Grading papers and visiting with coworkers minimizes staff's ability to supervise. Greeting students as they enter the school or classroom can positively impact staff's relationship building with them.

• Staff should position themselves in the middle of hallway traffic patterns. This will force groups of students to disband as they pass the central position, and will increase the supervisor's ability to see what is going on.

• Staff should engage students in conversation. When students appear upset or angry, talking to them may help staff ascertain what is wrong and to intervene, if appropriate.

• Staff should monitor restrooms near the area they supervise. Restrooms are high on the list of locations where inappropriate behavior occurs. High faculty visibility will discourage problem behavior.

• Staff should watch exterior doors that may be located near classrooms for unauthorized people entering or students exiting without permission. All staff members must be part of the access control plan for the school.

- Staff should watch for visitors or students who are not displaying—or who do not have—the necessary pass or badge. The value of visitor check-in procedures is greatly diminished if staff members do not speak with people who fail to follow the procedure.

- Staff should use hallway passes and classroom sign-out ledgers to help ensure that students are in the right place at the right time. A teacher's responsibility for student safety extends to the activities associated with giving them permission to leave class.

Handbooks should be specific and clear about supervision.

Now, take a minute to locate and review the teacher handbook for your school. Does it specifically address supervision? What guidance is provided for staff, and are expectations clear? If the handbook makes only a general statement that staff is expected to be in the hallways during class changes, then it probably does not provide enough direction, and school personnel will be left to interpret the administrative expectations and guidelines. **Remember, adult presence alone does not mean that students are adequately supervised.** Finally, check to see if the handbook references members of the support staff. As school employees, these important individuals have the responsibility for supervising students, if only indirectly and within the parameters of their assignments. If this responsibility has not been conveyed to the support staff, that oversight should be addressed.

PROVIDE APPROPRIATE STAFF DEVELOPMENT

In addition to issuing staff members a handbook that provides definition and guidance for student supervision, related staff development must be provided during the initial faculty meeting at the start of each school year.

- Within a few days of receiving the handbook, staff should be required to sign, indicating they have read and understood it, and that they have had an opportunity to ask questions.

- An administrator should retain agendas that provide documentation of items discussed in faculty meetings.

- Provisions should be made to ensure that substitute teachers and staff members hired after the beginning of the school year understand their supervisory responsibilities. Substitute teacher folders should include instructions for those teachers to follow the same supervisory guidelines as the regular teacher.

MODEL AND DISCUSS APPROPRIATE SUPERVISORY BEHAVIORS

The value of supervision cannot be overemphasized, and staff should be reminded of those expectations periodically throughout the school year. This can be accomplished through email messages, staff newsletters, posters in faculty lounges, and follow-up discussions at faculty meetings. Administrators should remember that ensuring understanding is not about telling someone something once. Rather, it is about teaching teachers how to accomplish the art of supervision while maintaining an atmosphere that is positive and conducive to learning.

Administrators should model proper supervisory techniques by refraining from personal adult conversations while they are on supervision duty. When faculty members see administrators who are not paying attention to students while on duty, they get the message that this is an acceptable practice.

Now, take a minute to think about the following questions:

• How does your school promote supervision and remind staff that it is an essential safe school strategy?

• Does your administrative team model appropriate supervisory techniques?

• What strategies do you currently have in place to inform substitute teachers and newly hired staff about the administrative expectations for supervision?

• Do you maintain yearly documentation related to staff development on the topic of supervision?

SUPERVISION MUST BE STRATEGIC TO BE EFFECTIVE

It's really not about working harder—it's about working smarter. Ask a fisherman what determines where the best place is to fish, and you are likely to hear about data analysis. It will probably include time of day, weather conditions, geography, first-hand experience, and fishing reports. A fisherman would not just randomly cast a line any more than a staff member should randomly decide where to supervise. While developing the supervisory plan, school personnel should review information such as disciplinary referrals, altercations, and faculty and student perceptions.

The strategic part of supervision is having a written plan and communicating it to those who are expected to carry out their duties. For most schools, one plan will not fit all. For some regularly occurring events and activities—such as arrival, dismissal, bus loading, lunch, and assemblies—a separate written plan should be devised, and then disseminated to those involved in supervisory roles. These written plans should include the following information:

- Beginning and ending times for supervisory duties
- Communication procedures, such as a requirement to carry a two-way radio or cell phone
- Unique or specific rules for the event being supervised
- Procedures and requirements for substitutions when supervising staff is absent
- Instructions for evacuations or in-place sheltering
- Expectations and duties for staff members
- Notations of special problems or areas requiring extra attention

TAKE STRATEGIC SUPERVISION INTO ACCOUNT WHEN PLANNING FOR NEW CONSTRUCTION OR REMODELING

New construction and building renovations provide opportunities for school personnel to increase the effectiveness of strategic supervision. To the extent that it is practical, avoid constructing hallways that are narrow or that contain protrusions, alcoves, or other features that may obstruct the supervising staff's view. Restrooms and other locations that are conducive to inappropriate student behavior should be located and designed with supervision in mind. The same applies to student centers and areas where large numbers of students congregate before and after school.

Soft drink machines and other large objects should be recessed into walls. Locating reception, secretarial, and other offices near where students assemble provides additional indirect supervision. The use of camera systems should be considered but should not replace staff presence. Landscaping and the placement of sidewalks and parking lots around the school affect pedestrian traffic patterns and change how students can be supervised. As personnel review construction plans, they should consider the plan's impact on supervision.

Maintaining a safe school environment requires implementing a number of proven strategies. Strategic supervision—which includes all staff members actively monitoring students and visitors to prevent safety lapses—should be at the top of every school administrator's list.

STRATEGY 4

A Safety Game Plan for Cocurricular Events

Staff members who oversee, direct, or coach cocurricular activities spend countless hours working and practicing with students—not only to ensure a top-quality performance, but also to ensure that the activities project a positive and polished image of the school. Whether it is a drama teacher preparing for a theatrical production, a coach developing a game plan for an upcoming competition, or a music teacher practicing with students for a PTA performance, everyone must understand that planning for the unexpected is a necessary part of the safety process.

When something goes awry at a cocurricular activity, there are a number of circumstances that can negatively affect safety in an already unusual situation. Consequently, school employees should give due diligence to planning for security at cocurricular activities throughout the school year by considering the following recommendations:

• A clear and structured chain of command for supervision should be in place. Indecision can be detrimental to successfully resolving or responding to an emergency situation. It is essential for all staff members who are working at a cocurricular activity to know who is assigned specific duties and where each person can be located in case of an emergency.

• Staff members acting in a supervisory role at cocurricular events should have adequate training, and should understand the expectations for making decisions. The administrator may not always be present at every after-school activity. In fact, it is not uncommon for teachers or other staff to be in charge at low-profile or lightly attended evening events. Nevertheless, the public expects the administrative designee to be as qualified and knowledgeable on safety-related issues as the principal or other administrators. Therefore, developing a handbook or checklist for those in charge of an event can be a real asset, especially for staff members who only occasionally find themselves in an administrative role. It is particularly important for those staff members to understand that they have the authority to make decisions.

• A meeting of staff members who are assigned to supervise or work the activity should be held before each cocurricular activity. This does not need to be a long or formal meeting, but it should review the specific duties and responsibilities of staff members and explain where supervisory staff members will be located during the event. In addition, the discussion topics should include how to contact or locate those in charge, how to handle any potential or anticipated problems, and how to verify that safety and security devices or supplies are readily available and working properly. In an emergency, staff members will be under stress and will be more likely to remember important information if it has been recently discussed.

• Evacuation routes and in-place sheltering locations should be identified, verified, and posted in clear view at all entrances and exits. When considering the location of sheltering areas, the anticipated size of the crowd should be considered. The maximum allowable occupancy should be posted at the entry to gymnasiums, auditoriums, or other locations where significant numbers of people attend school functions. When large crowds are expected, someone should be designated to monitor attendance to ensure that the maximum occupancy is not exceeded.

• In-place sheltering and evacuation maps should be developed that are specific to the locations that are commonly used for cocurricular events. Normal school-day sheltering and evacuation routes and maps usually reflect a student body that is spread throughout the building or campus, but that will not be the case at cocurricular activities. Consequently, plans specific to those locations should be developed. Be sure to include cafetoriums and food courts when developing evacuation and sheltering plans.

• It is advisable to announce certain safety information in advance of large events or when the noise level may be a serious factor in communicating with the crowd. For certain events, many schools already make announcements concerning tobacco usage, crowd conduct expectations, and so on. It is recommended that these announcements also contain information related to emergency exits and evacuation procedures. In addition, rules and conduct expectations should be posted at entryways to the events to remind everyone of what the school expects, condones, and prohibits.

• Supervisory staff members, ushers, or others who are designated to assist or oversee an event should wear easily recognizable attire. As part of the general announcements made at the beginning of an event, the crowd should be given instructions as to how to locate school staff members should the need arise. Staff who dress in apparel that display school colors or clothing with a mascot's image may tend to blend in with patrons and fans and may not be readily identified. It is therefore recommended that supervisory staff members wear badges that identify them as someone in authority. Wearing identical blazers, vests, or hats can also make staff members easy to identify, especially at events with large crowds.

• Staff members should be equipped with essential equipment and supplies, such as flashlights and cell phones. A small, powerful flashlight can be a valuable tool in the event of a power outage or if staff needs to go outside during evening hours to address a problem. In addition, staff should have a pocket-size notepad and pen; it is also a good practice for at least the supervisory staff to have cellular telephones. If two-way radios are used at the school, they should be carried by as many of the staff as is practical. Schools that are in areas where severe weather can be a threat should keep a weather-alert radio in a place where staff members will hear it if it is activated—perhaps in a concessions stand or ticket booth. For outside events, lightning detectors are also recommended.

• First aid supplies and emergency response kits should be located in the area where an event is being held. Although many athletic events will have a trainer or other similarly qualified person present, other cocurricular activities will not. Staff members should be aware of who among them has first aid training and where first aid supplies can be located. An emergency response kit should always be placed in areas where large numbers of students or the public congregate. In addition to the standard supplies that these kits normally contain, a battery-powered megaphone is recommended. This will be an invaluable tool if it is necessary to communicate to large numbers of people under adverse conditions.

• Local law enforcement agencies should be kept informed when large crowds are anticipated at cocurricular activities and events. Most law enforcement agencies are more than willing to disseminate a schedule of the school's events to the officer who covers that beat. Police departments like to be proactive and will want to know when large numbers are expected to attend a cocurricular activity. In addition to your scheduled staffing for security, having a police officer make a pass through the event or the school parking lots adds to the overall security plan for the event.

• Finally, scenario-based training should be provided to members of the crisis management team and others who may be called on to work cocurricular activities. School personnel should already be using tabletop exercises to train their school population about safety issues. Tabletop exercises are recommended by the U.S. Department of Education and are an excellent training method for a school's staff development program related to emergency response procedures. Consequently, it is recommended that personnel occasionally select a tabletop exercise where something is going awry at a cocurricular event. Forcing individuals to respond to the unusual circumstances of these events will allow for a better response when staff members and students are confronted with an actual emergency.

No school administrator can be at all activities, so training others to occasionally fill that role is critical. In the words of Ronald Reagan, "Surround yourself with the best people you can find, delegate authority, and don't interfere as long as the overall policy that you've decided on is being carried out."

STRATEGY 5

On the Road Again

Discipline Investigations Away From School

How prepared are you to manage the discipline, safety, and legal issues that occur on out-of-town, school-sponsored trips? To manage disciplinary incidents that occur in a school, personnel must know how to conduct an investigation, and must be familiar with the educational and statutory laws governing the procedural guidelines that must be followed. However, disciplinary issues will sometimes arise when students and staff are on school-sponsored activities that take them out of town, out of state, and—on rare occasions—out of the country. To avoid problems, administrators should address potential discipline issues, in advance, when the trip is being planned.

Besides disciplinary matters, accidents and injuries may also occur on out-of-town trips. Parents expect the school to have considered all contingencies and will insist staff members respond appropriately and decisively if an incident occurs. The following are some tips that should be followed prior to out-of-town trips:

• Checklists. Perhaps the best tool to assist staff with the safety planning process is to provide a written checklist of tasks to be completed prior to departure. The checklist should be considered a living document that can be modified by staff on their return, and used to prepare for future out-of-town events. A completed checklist should be part of the pretrip documentation record. When applicable, certain tasks on the list should include a time line for completion (see Resources).

• Trip handbooks. Expectations of behavior and the potential school and legal consequences should be discussed with students prior to trip departure. This information should be clearly communicated in a student handbook or a similar document designed for each specific trip. It should be reviewed with parents in a pretrip group meeting. After reviewing the document, parents and students should sign the document to acknowledge they have read and understood it.

• Laws of foreign countries. When the trip involves travel to a foreign country, parents and students should be reminded that the legal system in other countries may be very different from the U.S. legal system, and penalties may be much harsher—especially those related to the possession or use of controlled substances.

• Inspection of student belongings. Travel permission documents should give administrators the right to inspect a student's personal belongings prior to departure and at any time during the trip. When inspections are done randomly, they may negate the need for the threshold of reasonable suspicion usually required for a student search, though you should always consult legal counsel before including such language. We also suggest using the term "inspect" rather than "search." The word "search" may have additional legal implications, depending on local judicial interpretations. To ensure that the scope and nature of the inspections are appropriate, a set of written guidelines should be used, and more than one staff member should be present during the inspection. Only authorized staff members should be involved if there is a need to conduct an inspection of student belongings.

• Volunteer chaperones. When an administrative designee, in lieu of an administrator, is placed in charge of an out-of-town trip, the designee should have a thorough understanding of the disciplinary procedures and investigative requirements. When an administrator is left to handle an incident that occurred several days earlier across state lines, it may be difficult to reconstruct the circumstances if the incident was not handled properly at the time. Incorrect or inappropriate actions by chaperones who are not school employees may significantly hinder an administrator's ability to reconstruct an incident.

• Student handbooks and statement forms. Staff members on out-of-town trips should always take a copy of the student handbook and other documents that contain the discipline code; they should also take witness-statement forms. In most situations, it is not advisable to wait until after students return from a trip to take written and oral statements. The best statements are taken when an incident is fresh in everyone's mind and when there has not been an opportunity for those involved to compare stories, discuss the event, or collaborate.

• Cameras to document evidence. Chaperones for out-of-town trips should have a camera at their disposal for those circumstances when evidence will not be available at a later time, or where property damage has occurred. Pictures may be important evidence to document an event or a specific item. Cameras should be provided by the district to avoid any issues over the possession rights of the pictures.

• Local and state jurisdictions. Many states have statutes that require schools to notify law enforcement officials when certain types of offenses occur. Some state laws require schools to report certain types of incidents to the agency that has jurisdiction for that type of infraction. If in doubt, contact the police where the incident occurred and make the appropriate inquiries related to state and municipal regulations. Obtain a copy of the written police report if one is prepared. If the police counsel no action, ask the officer to put that counsel in writing.

- Dealing with contraband. Law enforcement officials should be contacted when contraband, such as controlled substances or weapons, is seized. Maintaining possession of these items until the return to the home school is risky and may be illegal. However, pictures of the contraband should be taken as part of the record of events.

- Debriefing. In the aftermath of a serious incident occurring on an out-of-town trip, it is important for staff members and those directly involved with the incident to debrief as a group. This will provide two valuable sources of information: First, depending on the level of media involvement and the seriousness of the event, debriefing will provide the administrator with the best overall picture of the who, what, where, when, how, and why of the incident. Second, debriefing provides an opportunity to adjust the planning process for the next out-of-town trip.

Taking students to school-sponsored activities and letting them participate in out-of-town cocurricular trips is a valuable and viable part of any comprehensive school experience. If school personnel have already made proper preparations during the planning process, discipline violations, accidents, and injuries that occur on out-of-town trips can be managed successfully. Remember: prior to an out-of-town event, it is important to clearly communicate all of a school's behavioral and procedural expectations with parents, students, accompanying staff members, and chaperones. Should a regrettable incident occur, administrators will be better prepared to act quickly, decisively, and appropriately.

STRATEGY 6

Visitor Check-in and Screening Procedures

It's More Than Just Signing the Visitor Log

Systematic and consistent check-in and screening procedures for school visitors help ensure the safety of the school environment. Although a visitor check-in system is a standard operating procedure for most school buildings, establishing systematic, practical, and successful visitor check-in and screening procedures entails much more than making visitors sign a visitor's log and giving them an identification badge. To implement a successful visitor check-in process, staff members must first have a clear understanding of the need for check-in procedures. The real purpose of visitor check-in and screening procedures is not only to observe and identify individuals who have followed the procedures, but also to make it easier to identify those individuals who have not followed them.

POSTING CHECK-IN PROCEDURES

All entry points to the school should have the rules and procedures for visitor check-in clearly posted. It is recommended these be written in both English and Spanish. Posting the rules serves two purposes: First, it provides an opportunity to notify visitors that they will be required to follow established procedures when they visit the school. Second, it provides the basis for inquiry when staff members must confront individuals who have disregarded the posted instructions.

Individuals who arrive at the school without the intention to engage in prohibited behavior will generally follow visitor check-in procedures. However, those arriving to do otherwise will, in most situations, disregard the posted instructions.

PROCEDURE

School secretaries often feel embarrassed when they are checking in a visitor who is well known within the school community, but all staff members should understand that an important aspect of successful access control is maintaining consistency in administering procedures. Listed below are some specific strategies that should be considered when setting up or reviewing your school's current visitor screening and check-in procedure.

• Signage. Instructions that clearly portray visitor check-in requirements and direct visitors to the proper check-in location should be posted at all entry points. If a local ordinance or other legal requirement is the basis for enforcement, the signage should so indicate.

• Screening requirements. Additional signage should appear at the check-in location to advise visitors that school staff members reserve the right to ask for picture identification. Visitor check-in and screening requirements should also appear in student handbooks and in school newsletters that are sent home. The goal is to provide as much advanced notice of the check-in and screening procedures as possible. This will usually result in greater compliance within the school community.

• Friendly conversation. As part of the standard check-in procedure, the staff member on duty should engage each visitor in a friendly conversation to determine if there are any abnormalities in the visitor's demeanor or mental state. This provides an opportunity to ascertain if the individual is unhappy or agitated with staff members or students, or if the individual is under the influence of a controlled substance.

• Visitor log. The visitor log should indicate who the visitor is, the reason for the visit, the person the visitor will be seeing, and the times the visitor checks in and out. The staff member who processes the visitor's check-in should initial the visitor log; having staff members take ownership of this process will ensure greater attention to detail.

• Legibility. Unless the staff member who is overseeing the check-in procedure recognizes the visitor, the visitor's signature should be checked for legibility. If the signature is unreadable, the staff member should ask the visitor to pronounce the name.

• Picture identification. The decision to ask for picture identification should be based on the comfort level the staff member has regarding whether the visitor is, in fact, who he or she claims to be. Staff members should always err on the side of caution and request identification if there is any doubt.

• Visitor badges. Visitor badges should be color coded, numbered, and designed so individuals who fail to return their badges on leaving the campus cannot readily use the same badge on another day. Moreover, reusable badges should be inventoried periodically to ensure that they are all accounted for and ready for use. Commercially produced visitor badges that are designed for one-time use are also available. It makes little sense to design a secure check-in procedure if the visitor can leave with a badge that can be reused another day.

- Staff notification. When a visitor arrives, it is a good idea to alert the person who is receiving the visitor. This can provide the staff member at the time of check-in with additional information if the visitor is someone who may be expected to create a problem. For added security, staff members may want to escort visitors through the school to the meeting or classroom.

TRAINING AND PREPARATION

The final part of a sound visitor check-in procedure is to ensure all staff members understand the process and their role in the overall success of the program. The person assigned to process visitors is only one part of the procedure. The rest of the staff should act as eyes and ears within the building or on the campus, and be aware of any persons who ignore the check-in process, are intent on creating a disruption, or might pose a threat to the school population.

Staff members who check visitors in should receive a written copy of the school's building or campus procedures, as well as instructions about how to respond when a visitor is noncompliant or exhibits unusual behavior. All staff should receive training in how to approach and tactfully engage in dialogue with individuals who do not have visitor identification badges. These instructions should include information about how to properly respond to a visitor's defiant or abusive behavior. A friendly demeanor can sometimes defuse even the angriest person. When that does not work, staff should remain calm, speak softly, keep a reasonable distance, and stand at a right angle when speaking with the individual. However, if the visitor is visibly agitated and distressed, the staff member should get to the nearest communication device and notify the office of the visitor's presence and location on the campus.

Visiting a school campus can and should be a positive experience for everyone in the school community, and most of the time it is just that. Publicizing, practicing, and providing written procedures for staff to follow when visitors arrive should be a routine part of each school year. Visitor check-in requirements can then be accurately promoted as one of the components that a school uses to ensure a safe environment.

STRATEGY 7

Ensuring the Safe Evacuation of Students With Physical Disabilities During an Emergency

For in-place sheltering and evacuation plans to work during an emergency, schools need to prepare—and practice—individualized evacuation and shelter plans for students with disabilities.

Throughout the school year, students and staff participate in fire drills and severe weather drills that are usually simple and routine. But what happens when a school cannot accommodate students with physical disabilities through the normal sheltering and evacuation procedures? Just as schools are committed to meeting the educational requirements of students with physical disabilities, schools should be committed to develop a plan to evacuate and shelter in place these students during an emergency event.

Because of the unique risks and circumstances associated with moving students who have limited mobility or complete immobility, administrators should take the following factors into consideration when making evacuation plans:

- Physical conditions that may create additional risks for students with disabilities if they have to be moved rapidly
- Special equipment or medication that must accompany students with disabilities
- The use of stairways, as opposed to elevators, during an evacuation
- Evacuation routes that require students to traverse terrain that could be affected by bad weather
- Evacuations that may require students and staff to travel a considerable distance to be clear of the danger
- The assignment of staff members to assist students with special needs during evacuation and in-place sheltering
- The supervision of students whose teachers have been temporarily reassigned to assist students with physical disabilities
- The special circumstances associated with cocurricular activities and events—such as crowd movement—and the availability of sheltering locations and evacuation routes from auditoriums, gymnasiums, and stadiums
- Special considerations for students with physical disabilities who may also have emotional and cognitive impairments

- Schedule and class modifications made throughout the school year that will affect the location of students with physical disabilities during the school day
- Classrooms that, by their specific design, cannot be relocated to a ground level

DEVELOPING AN INDIVIDUALIZED EVACUATION AND SHELTERING PLAN

Every student with a disability who could be adversely affected during an evacuation or in-place sheltering event should have an individualized evacuation and sheltering plan (IESP). The IESP should be an addendum to the school's emergency response plan and should include the following:

- The class schedules of students with disabilities
- Information about any specific medical conditions of students with disabilities, including notations about medications and critical peripheral equipment such as the need for an oxygen tank or wheelchair
- Any special instructions on medically approved techniques for the physical movement of a student with a disability, such as restrictions for lifting, and so on
- A sheltering location in close proximity to each of the classrooms used by students with disabilities
- A designated exterior exit for evacuation and an alternate exit specific to each class that a student with a disability attends
- Staff members and alternates who are assigned to assist in the evacuation or in-place sheltering of students with disabilities

Written operating instructions for medical equipment should accompany the student.

The school nurse, students, parents, and an administrator should all provide input into the IESP process and sign the document when it has been completed to indicate they have reviewed and agreed. In some cases, it may also be well advised to consult the physicians of students with disabilities. Members of the emergency response team should have a copy of the IESP as an addendum to their individual emergency response plans. In addition, any classroom teacher who has daily or periodic responsibility for a student with a disability should have a copy of the student's IESP. The plan should also be given to persons involved in the actual transport of students with disabilities. A copy of the IESP should also be included in the folder provided to substitute teachers.

PRACTICING THE IESP

Writing the IESP is only the first step in the process. The IESP is of little value until it has been practiced and modified as appropriate. When school personnel practice evacuation and in-place sheltering plans for students with disabilities, the following considerations should be taken into account:

• School personnel involved in assisting students with disabilities should clearly understand each student's medical condition. When possible, parents should be encouraged to observe a practice drill. By doing so, they will be able to provide input and will have a greater comfort level with the process.

• When possible, use the same staff members each time a student with a disability is moved. When possible, assign alternate staff members to fill this role in the event the primary staff member is absent. Transporting these students might not be an easy task. Consequently, both designees and alternates should be trained in how to correctly transport a physically disabled student so neither staff nor student safety is compromised.

• It may be ill advised to physically carry a student with a disability during a practice evacuation drill. However, the student should be present during the drill so the student will understand the proper procedure. When necessary, a mannequin or dummy can be used during a practice drill; the local fire department is a good resource for obtaining such an item. Staff members who are assigned to move students should be reminded that these individuals may have limited movement in some limbs and may be unable to protect themselves during a fall.

• Evacuation plans should account for times when students with disabilities are not in a classroom, such as during lunch or class changes. In addition, students with disabilities should be told what actions they should take if something happens during times when they are not with a staff member.

• Remember that a student with a disability may not be able to assume protective positions during certain in-place sheltering events, such as during earthquakes or severe weather. Therefore, it is important for administrators to work with local emergency management officials and district risk management staff members to identify where and how these students should be protected.

• Use monthly drill reports to note when practice sessions involving students with disabilities occurred. This information is an important part of any school's routine record keeping.

• Remember to debrief relevant participants after all practice and actual evacuations. Although debriefing should be an integral part of crisis planning, it is often overlooked because of time constraints.

ASSISTING STUDENTS WITH SHORT-TERM PHYSICAL NEEDS

Throughout the school year, there will be students with temporary medical conditions, such as a broken leg, who will have restricted mobility. Consequently, a short-term IESP will need to be considered. An appointed staff member should have the responsibility for monitoring and updating all evacuation plans for these students. The school nurse might be a good person for this task.

Although practice drills are an invaluable tool in preparing to evacuate a student with a disability, administrators should remember there are certain factors—panic, stress, and so on—that will be present in an actual event that cannot be simulated in a practice drill. Although perfection is seldom achieved in the world of school safety, thorough planning and regular practice will certainly be a means toward that end.

Authors' note: As is true in life, many valuable lessons are learned through experience. As readers you might be interested to know the information shared within this article is a direct result of a fire drill involving a physically disabled student that went awry. While it was true there was a plan, it was not detailed enough and did not account for the absence of one of the designated transporters. Thus, the idea of an IESP had its inception. It was a valuable lesson learned for all involved.

STRATEGY 8

Invest in a Safety Committee

Creating Strategies You Can Bank On

A safety committee requires time, energy, and sometimes money, but the rewards can be significant. Call it a focus group, a team, a commission, or a board, but a committee by any other name is still a committee. And isn't it just what everyone needs? Ah yes, another committee to monitor, chair, and facilitate. Right? Absolutely not! But before the idea of adding to an already overstressed workload makes you stop reading, please consider the fact that taking the time to institute a productive school safety committee will ultimately be time well spent in terms of shared expertise, professional and personal liability, and overall schoolwide safety. Does that sound like it has some possibilities? Of course it does.

Often underutilized, a school safety committee is one of the best tools an administrator can have. If formed carefully, this group can help create, maintain, and assess school safety and climate in a strategic, intentional, and timely manner throughout the school year.

It is virtually impossible for any one person to be solely responsible for the safety and security needs of elementary, middle, and high school students and staff in the twenty-first century. Schools that have a positive and safe educational environment usually have it because all staff contributes to ensuring it. In fact, if a school's overall safety plans do not encourage—or require—the participation of staff from all departments, the plans will be compromised.

A safety committee will encourage staff member participation through a multidisciplinary mix of members. This combination is necessary if the committee is to be effective. Bringing together individuals who have expertise in specific areas and a vested interest in a safe and secure work environment will pay big dividends over time.

WHO ARE THE PLAYERS?

When forming a committee designed to facilitate safety and security, school personnel will want to ensure the right players are included. The following are some of the areas, departments, and groups that should be represented:

- Administration
- Counseling

- Health
- Secretarial
- Security
- Food service
- Custodial and maintenance
- Teaching staff
- Athletic staff
- Student body

Depending on the composition, special considerations, or unique needs of the school, there may be other staff who also need to be a part of the school safety committee. Representatives from each of the listed areas will bring specific expertise and unique perspectives to the table. The mix of individuals from these various departments will broaden the knowledge base of all committee members, making them more effective and versatile in the event of an emergency.

WHAT IS THE PURPOSE?

Safety committees must operate with clear direction and purpose. "Safety" is too broad a term to simply designate it as the purpose. It is important for the committee to have well-defined functions and specific tasks. Creating a document that outlines these administrative expectations will help provide structure and guidance to the committee members.

WHAT ARE SOME SUGGESTED
DUTIES AND ACTIVITIES?

A frustration of many administrators is ensuring basic safety and security functions and strategies are consistently in place throughout the school. The larger the school, the more difficult this becomes. Safety committees can develop guidelines and ensure compliance by developing checklists that are completed by each staff member in the school. For example, the committee might consult with the school nurse to create a checklist of first aid supplies that should be readily available in each classroom. In turn, each teacher would verify once each semester that the supplies are available in the assigned area and note such on a copy of the checklist. This process creates the kind of participatory leadership imperative to any school safety plan. The same process can be used to verify that evacuation and sheltering plans are posted, door locks are in working order, important telephone numbers are posted, and so forth (see Resources).

WHAT SHOULD BE DONE FIRST?

Certainly a good place to start is a review of accident statistics and data. The committee can and should review each accident, and should examine statistical and anecdotal information to identify possible causation. Then the committee will be able to recommend actions to reduce the likelihood of a recurrence. The committee should also follow up, and periodically review that the recommended actions have been implemented.

A well-chosen and energized safety committee may prevent a significant number of accidents. Developing schoolwide themes, projects, and initiatives will enhance the overall safety of the school, and will create and maintain a high level of awareness among staff and students. Tackling such issues as thefts at school by providing information to students and staff on how to avoid becoming a victim will help address that problem. There are a limitless number of activities and projects that can be used to enhance the safety of the school climate and environment.

WHAT IS THE COST?

The actual monetary expenditure of a safety committee is minimal, but some funds for supplies and materials may be necessary. It is not realistic to expect a safety committee not to recommend some strategies that have an associated cost or develop safety awareness promotional programs without some expenditure.

The question is, "What will the cost ultimately be if such a committee is not formed and fully functioning?" The fear of generating costly and untimely work orders should not be a reason to delay forming a safety committee. In matters such as school safety, timing is everything.

WHAT WILL BE THE RESULTS?

The value of a safety committee should be measured not only in the dollars and cents saved, but also in the benefit it provides in the area of academics. When a school increases its safety record, it will likely increase the feeling of safety, which will have positive effects on student and staff attendance, and on academic achievement. If a school experiences a tragedy or accident of significant consequence, staff and student emotions are affected long after the event. Safety can and does affect everyone, and safety is a fundamental need for all. When a school begins to experience a reduction in accidents, injuries, school crime, and disciplinary problems, personnel will spend less time with these issues and more time doing what is more rewarding and important—spending quality time with students.

STRATEGY 9

Speaking of School Safety

Creating a Conversation Within the School Community

Conversations about school safety should take place throughout the year to assure parents and community members that the school is prepared for emergencies.

Communicating with parents and others in the school community on the topic of school safety can be a balancing act. Say too little and parents may believe not enough is being done to address safety and security concerns. Say too much and some will assume personnel are overreacting or that the school has serious safety issues that need to be addressed by extreme measures. Either way, it takes reflection and insight on the part of school personnel to decide what to explain regarding safety and security measures and when it is appropriate to share information. It can be a win-win or a lose-lose situation, depending on the circumstances prompting the release of information, the interpretation of the information by the listener, and the ability of the school official to communicate clearly, strategically, succinctly, and confidently.

QUESTIONS FOR CONSIDERATION

Before considering how to share information about school safety, ask yourself the following questions:

- What type of information is appropriate to share?

- How detailed should the information be?

- In what format is this type of information best communicated?

- When is the best time for this type of information to be disseminated? Should it be a routine part of the beginning of a new school year, disseminated only in the aftermath of a tragic event, or a combination of both? We recommend being proactive, as opposed to being reactive, when it comes to making this decision.

- What board policies, if any, need to be considered?

Educators know the feeling of safety is essential to students and staff to maximize academic achievement and to recruit and retain employees.

Promoting school safety should be part of the school's routine, and discussing safety and security with parents and others in the community should be as important as promoting academics, cocurricular activities, special programs, and other services. Although there may be a few specific details of safety and security that are privileged information, such as bomb threat procedures and threat assessment screening, most strategies are already visible; their value will not be compromised if they are broadcast.

SEVEN POINTS TO SHARE

Seven topic areas we believe should be discussed as part of the routine dialogue are outlined in the following paragraphs. For emphasis and clarity, we provide suggested language.

• The school has a comprehensive emergency response plan. The plan is reviewed periodically and updated when necessary. Emergency procedures are practiced with the faculty, staff, and students. The school works closely with local emergency service providers to ensure everyone is prepared for an emergency. The school conducts drills for fire, severe weather events, and armed intruders.

• The school has a check-in procedure for visitors during the school day. Although we encourage parents to visit our campus, please keep in mind check-in procedures apply to all visitors as part of our access control measures. Visitors should use the appropriate entrance and be prepared to state the nature of their visit, sign a guest register, and show picture identification if asked to do so. Our procedures are structured to help ensure the safety of all students and staff. We ask that you set the correct example for others by following them.

• Parents should contact school personnel as quickly as possible if they become aware of a situation that could endanger students or staff members. As a parent, you are a valuable partner in helping us ensure a safe school environment. When you have any safety and security information the school should know, please contact a building administrator, school counselor, or teacher immediately. We will treat all information in an appropriately confidential manner.

• As a district, we have adopted a variety of safety and security policies, including a student code of conduct we enforce fairly and consistently. All students are provided a copy of the student code of conduct in the student handbook, which is also available online at the school's website. Parents are asked to read and review the handbook with their children. In addition, parents are welcome to contact school officials with their questions and concerns about content, implementation, or enforcement of school policies.

- We have procedures in place for disseminating information to parents and the greater community during an emergency. In the case of an emergency in the community, listen to local radio and television stations. This information will also be posted on the district's website and sent electronically via text message to cell phones and email addresses, as provided by the parents. As quickly as possible, we will provide information on how, where, and when parents can pick up their children. In some emergencies, it may not be advisable for you to come to the school. Please remember the safety of your children is foremost in our minds, and you may be required to show identification as an added security measure before your child is released to you. If the school is considered by law enforcement to be a crime scene, students will not be released until the police instruct school officials to do so.

- We use the expertise of a school safety team throughout the school year. Although injuries and disciplinary infractions occur periodically, all necessary precautions are taken to ensure the school environment remains hazard free. Our school safety team includes administrators, the school nurse, a counselor, a custodian, a member of the food service staff, and selected teachers. The team routinely reviews accident reports and discipline violations to determine whether adjustments must be made to supervision policies, the student code of conduct, or the school building. Please contact the school if you believe you have information about a safety hazard.

- Our school uses a number of strategies to help ensure a safe climate. The following is a sample of what we do to help ensure a safe learning environment for students and staff members:
  - A nurse and a school counselor are available during the school day.
  - Specific procedures for supervision are in place.
  - Visitors are required to follow check-in procedures.
  - Students and staff members are required to wear identification badges.
  - A school resource officer is assigned to the campus.
  - Coaches and certain selected staff members have first aid and CPR training.
  - Surveillance cameras are placed strategically throughout the campus.
  - Volunteers greet students in the morning as they arrive.
  - Peer mediation and conflict resolution teams are available to students.
  - An antiviolence curriculum is incorporated in lessons throughout the year.
  - The discipline code is enforced consistently.
  - Custodial staff members routinely check doors and grounds throughout the school day.

CONCLUSION

Remember, parents, students, and the entire school community should be involved in maintaining a safe learning environment. Teachers do not mention an important concept only once and expect every student to internalize and understand it. To truly teach is to repeatedly explain and reinforce what others need to know. Although the conversation about safety may begin at a meeting with parents in September, the topic should be part of the overall message from the school throughout the year.

For most people, it is enough to know the school staff is making every effort to address safety and security concerns, but the community will not be aware of that if it is not communicated clearly and often. Host parent meetings, use the school's website, or provide information through the school newsletter—or do all three. Just keep parents informed.

STRATEGY 10

Closing Out the School Year

Every school leader approaches the month of May and the subsequent end-of-year tasks with mixed feelings of stress and relief.

Although preparations for ensuring a safe ending to the school year are crucial, for many schools the month of May will also be a time for transition from the regular school year into a summer school program or other activities. End-of-year tasks are important, but it is important not to overlook what must be readied for these summer activities as well as beginning the preparation for the next school year.

A number of items should be on a "To Do" list related to school and student safety as the regular school year concludes, including the following:

1. Identify students who planned to graduate but who will not do so because of academic issues or discipline violations that occur at the end of the school year. Staff should be kept informed of these students; not being allowed to participate in graduation ceremonies can be a triggering event for violent or escalating aggressive behavior. Principals, counselors, and parents should maintain dialogue with the student and monitor the student's mental state. In addition, an effort should be made to ascertain if the student plans to attend the graduation ceremony. When practical, it is recommended pictures of these students be provided at graduation ceremonies to security and other supervisory staff who may not recognize them by sight.

2. Encourage teachers and other staff to remain vigilant for students who exhibit signs of threatening behavior. This directive should come in the form of a written reminder and should be reinforced at end-of-year faculty meetings. Supervision does not end until the last student leaves the campus on the last day of school.

3. Remember that access control is basic and critical to maintaining safety within a school. End-of-year activities will create additional visitors to the campus as well as greater student movement to and from the school. Consequently, access control can be even more frustrating for administrators; vigilance by all must be maintained. Inconvenience to staff or a patron is not a reason to ignore established visitor check-in procedures. If you are expecting an influx of patrons for an end-of-year assembly, make several staff members available at school entrances to issue visitor identification badges.

4. Plan carefully for field trips, school picnics, and senior excursions. During the end of the year, many types of student activities are scheduled. Make certain there are sufficient chaperones when students are taken out of their familiar environments. Students should understand the parameters for exploration, and should be allowed to participate only after parents have given written permission for them to do so. If the length of the school day is shortened, make certain this information is provided in a variety of formats to parents prior to the early dismissal days.

5. Provide adequate security and supervision at such end-of-year functions as proms and graduation ceremonies. It is important to clearly set and communicate expectations to both students and staff. It is also advisable to provide the local law enforcement agency with a listing of the end-of-year activities where large crowds are expected. In many jurisdictions, local law enforcement officers may be instructed to put these events on special patrol.

6. Explore the possibility of using private security for the evening and overnight hours during the last few weeks of school. Many schools experience an increase in vandalism at the end of the school year. In lieu of hiring outside services or to supplement such, consider adjusting custodial work shifts to create an overnight presence on the campus. At a minimum, ask local law enforcement to patrol the campus more frequently as the school year comes to a close.

7. Account for all building and room keys at the end of the school year and collect them from the staff and faculty who will not be returning in the fall. Also collect district identification badges, parking permits, and other items issued to employees. If the school utilizes an intrusion alarm system, make sure that access privileges have been removed for nonreturning staff and faculty.

8. Move mobile electronic equipment from rooms not in use during the summer months to an area of high security during that time period. Valuable items should not be left near windows or exterior doors for extended times when school is not in session. For schools that have intrusion alarm systems, equipment should be placed where alarm coverage is available and practical. An inventory of major equipment should be completed at the beginning and end of the summer months. As part of the "check-out procedure," individual classroom teachers should complete the end-of-year inventory specific to the classroom.

9. Start planning for the next school year in terms of safety and security. Although the school year is coming to an end, it is not too early to begin thinking about safety and security for the next school year. As part of one of the last faculty meetings it is a good idea to spend a

designated amount of time debriefing the staff and compiling a list of the things related to staff and student safety to be done differently during the next school year. Some of the items discussed may require work orders or specific modifications which will need to be completed over the summer months. With the window of opportunity consisting of only a few months, it will be important to plan how these tasks will be accomplished. The summer will also provide the opportunity to address those items from the debriefing list that are procedural in nature, which may require changes in handbooks, directives, or postings and placards.

10. Review the exterior lighting and other environmental issues such as foliage around the school. As foliage increases in size with each passing year, it can begin to create shadowing and negate the value of the intended lighting schemes. At the end of the school year and throughout the summer months, lighting takes on an added significance. Check that all lighting is functioning and is illuminating the intended areas.

11. Review the close of school year issues with staff related to safety and security. Because this task takes time, making a checklist for individuals to follow will help ensure that important items are not forgotten. In addition, assigning specific tasks to department heads, custodial staff, secretarial staff, and teaching staff will serve three purposes. First, it will help with the already full schedule of end-of-year "must do's." Second, it will create ownership because the entire staff is taking part in specific tasks. Third, it will continually reinforce the need to put safety and security at the forefront as the school year concludes.

12. Visitor check-in procedures and other security strategies related to movement of individuals in and out of the building should be continued. While summer school or other activities generally bring with them fewer disciplinary issues, the overall issue of building security is not lessened. Administrators should also make certain summer school students are provided with pertinent information such as student handbooks and codes of conduct, and that they are afforded the opportunity to practice emergency drills.

13. A concerted effort should be made to familiarize summer school staff and students to the specific procedures and practices within the summer school sites. Often, staff and students are assigned to schools that are not their regular assignments. In an emergency, staff and students will respond to the way they have practiced and planned. Therefore, acclimating staff and students to the new environment will be crucial. This procedure should include practicing evacuation and in-place sheltering drills.

PROACTIVE MEASURES

Planning for safety and security is critical in minimizing the chances that an unpleasant or tragic event will occur at the close to the school year or during the summer months. While every day of a school year has the potential to generate a number of safety and security issues, the end of a school year creates unique circumstances that must be considered as part of the cycle of planning and preparation for student and staff safety.

2

Response Strategies

STRATEGY 11

Planning for School Emergencies: Part 1

Regardless of what many people believe, educators know schools are not dormant during the summer months. In addition to scheduling special learning activities, working on building renovations, and planning for the next school year, summer is an ideal time to reflect on and update the school's emergency response plan. A school has safety obligations all year, but these obligations are elevated when students arrive on the first day of the school year. Staff should review the school's emergency preparations before that first day of school. The first part of a two-part plan, Strategy 11 provides tips and information to help principals and staff members review and update the school's emergency response plan.

A MULTILEVEL PLAN

There are various levels of emergency planning that take place in any community. Each level is interwoven with the next level, culminating with plans developed at the national level. For school personnel, emergency planning starts with the classroom and progresses upward through the school and district plans. Segments developed for the local community should fit into the overall plan.

Classroom Plans

Every teacher should be asked to view the classroom as a separate school environment and to have a plan in place for ensuring the safety of the students under direct supervision. A relatively simple written outline of this plan should be easy to access. A flip chart is one of the most easily used formats for an emergency response plan.

Placed in a location where it can be quickly found, the flip chart should contain brief steps the teacher can follow to protect students from harm in emergency situations. Although sample flip charts can be commercially purchased, they should contain the events and response strategies that are part of the school's actual emergency response plan. The plans should include general sheltering and evacuation plans for the classroom as well as responses to fires, weather-related events, chemical or hazardous material leaks or spills, armed intruders, and other events that may require immediate action by the teacher.

School Plan

A school's emergency response plan should be a framework of such key functions as communications, evacuations, sheltering, and first aid. Although emergencies do not follow a script, all staff must know the basic components of the plan and be able to adapt each component to the circumstances accompanying a specific event. In a true emergency, staff members may not have time to find the plan and locate the page that tells them what they are supposed to do.

As a multifaceted document dealing with a variety of potential emergencies, the plan and its specific components should occasionally be reviewed by local emergency service providers. The outside review should be conducted by law enforcement officials, fire and emergency response teams, and disaster management officials.

The National Incident Management System (NIMS) is familiar to local emergency service providers, but it may be unfamiliar to school administrators. NIMS was created in 2004 by the U.S. Department of Homeland Security as the national standard for emergency and disaster planning. It is a structured system for command, control, and decision making when responding to various localized, regional, and national disasters. NIMS is in the implementation stage nationally and should be incorporated into school and district disaster and emergency plans. Local emergency service providers can help schools write a plan that incorporates NIMS.

District Plan

Every school district should have an emergency response plan that addresses how the district will support an individual school during and after an emergency, and how it will support multiple schools if the emergency is widespread. Each school administrator should be familiar with the district's plan and with the resources available if the school is directly or indirectly affected by a tragedy. Building-level administrators at schools that are not directly affected by an emergency event may become part of the district response team. The district may ask administrators whose schools are not affected by an emergency event to help the affected schools. For this reason, building-level school administrators should be thoroughly familiar with the district plan.

Community Plan

School administrators also should be familiar with how their school fits into the community disaster plan. In many communities, school buildings are designated as relocation or evacuation sites. There may be a need to house hundreds or thousands of individuals who are displaced because of a natural or manmade disaster, and this need may occur at a moment's notice. Also, schools in many parts of the country are designated as inoculation sites in the event of biological terrorism or an epidemic. Such events would significantly disrupt the school's routine or cause widespread school cancellations.

DEVELOPING YOUR PLAN

Although it is important to be familiar with all levels of planning discussed above, the building-level administrator is mainly held accountable for developing and overseeing an individual school's plan. Therefore, it is essential that principals ensure the school's emergency response plan is designed and written to be a usable reference and operational document under even the most difficult and extreme circumstances.

Plans are never written when the crisis response team is under stress; consequently, plans seldom reflect a worst-case-scenario thought process. Under stress, an individual's sensory perceptions undergo radical changes. The individual's ability to hear, see, feel, and smell are all altered. Respiration and heart rates increase, and multiple chemical changes occur in the body as a direct result of the level of stress the individual is experiencing. When assembling a safety plan, it is important to recognize that the individuals using the plan will most likely be under some level of stress.

Here are some tips to help develop a user-friendly and functional plan that can be helpful even under adverse conditions:

• Emergency plan documents should contain bulleted or short, direct statements wherever practical. When under stress, a person's ability to read and comprehend material written in lengthy sentences or paragraphs is significantly impaired. Sections that contain segmented material, such as those commonly found in assignments and duties and responsibilities, should be written using vertical columns that separate information by categories and use only brief wording (see Resources). Where feasible, use oversized fonts so written material is easier to see and read.

• Color-coding or flagging should be used for important information on maps and diagrams. Locating key information will be easier if it is easily distinguished from other items displayed.

• Plans should have a table of contents or index to help people quickly locate the information they need. In an emergency, seconds can be valuable.

• Individual components of the plan should be labeled as "critical" or "reference" documents and located in the appropriate section. In addition, each component of the plan should show the date it was last reviewed and last modified, as well as how many pages should be present for each particular document. This will make routine auditing of the plan easier.

• A three-ring binder works best for holding copies of the plan. Because notebooks around work areas are usually plentiful and sometimes hard to distinguish from one another, it is advisable to select a bright color that will stand out, and to label the binder's spine so it can be located quickly in an emergency.

• Emergency plans provided to the emergency response team should have plastic protectors for individual pages. This will help ensure their legibility in situations where water, debris, or other conditions would damage unprotected paper.

Clearly written and easily accessible guidelines will be essential in the event of an emergency or disaster. With a plan, you will be able to respond to any situation more quickly and effectively. Set aside some time to create or update such plans for your classrooms, school, and district. The next strategy, which is the second part of this two-part plan, examines specific documents that should be included in a school's plan for emergencies.

STRATEGY 12

Planning for School Emergencies: Part 2

In Strategy 11 (Part 1 of this two-part plan), we discussed the various types of emergency plans with which administrators should be familiar, and how each is interconnected in the event of a local or regional incident. We also provided tips for enhancing the school emergency plan to make it as user friendly as possible. However, because it is impossible to comprehensively cover all facets of an emergency plan, it is imperative school personnel stay well educated on this topic, review plans on a routine basis, and always plan in terms of worst-case scenarios.

COMMUNICATIONS COMPONENT

In many emergencies, administrators must decide whether the unfolding event warrants in-place sheltering or evacuation. There are a number of variables that affect not only whether to initiate one of these two actions, but also just how to accomplish the task. In many situations, the decision to shelter in place or evacuate must be made in a matter of seconds. It is for these and other reasons that communication plans for notifying students, staff, and faculty members should not use coded or veiled words. The following tips are valuable when writing this section of the plan.

Use Simple, Direct Language

Communication plans for in-place sheltering and evacuation should use simple yet direct language to communicate what students, staff, and faculty members, and others in the school should do. The NIMS planning model, which was discussed in Strategy 11, strongly encourages everyone to use straightforward language for issuing instructions, rather than using "coded" language (such as "Code Red," "Code Green," or a coded announcement such as, "The copier equipment repairman is in the building"). An inherent problem with using coded language is that, on a given day, individuals may be present who might not understand the code words being used. Straightforward language provides the best chance for people to understand what is expected of them and how they should act.

Use the Intercom Effectively

Students, staff, and faculty members are in a constant state of movement, and there will be a number of opportunities for any of these groups to be in places where normal communication is difficult. Band and choir rooms, industrial technology rooms, and gymnasiums and locker rooms are a few places where, depending on the activity in progress, intercom announcements may go unheard. It is important for communication plans to account for potential trouble areas through the use of alternative contact procedures. Depending on the situation, runners might be a viable option; for some in-place sheltering events, however, this may not be practical or safe. Consequently, other means will have to be built into the plan, such as the use of staff members in adjoining classrooms to assist in notification, or visual alerts for the classroom teacher, such as a flashing light near the intercom speaker.

Communication Is a Two-Way Process

Although verification that actions have been completed by teachers and other staff members may be vital in some circumstances, staff should wait to be contacted during an in-place sheltering event unless there is a compelling reason for them to initiate communication. Classrooms with only overhead public address speakers for communication may create a privacy issue for the teacher and administrator, and loud background noise could make communication difficult. We recommend that plans include alternative contact methods to allow for those circumstances.

During evacuations, especially evacuations of large campuses, staff may need to communicate with those in charge to report a problem, or to report that all students are or are not accounted for. Although two-way radios may be useful, hand or flag signals can also be used for rapid communication. Establishing a uniform set of procedures as part of the communication plan will facilitate the exchange of information. Administrators may find that a bullhorn or similar device is essential in communicating to large groups outdoors, or as an alternative communication device for indoors, depending on the circumstances. The ability to communicate is vital to maintaining order during an emergency.

EQUIPMENT AND SUPPLIES COMPONENT

Successfully navigating an emergency event is not only about having well-trained individuals in key positions, but also about having the necessary equipment, tools, and supplies available; knowing where they are located; and being familiar with their use.

Not all members of an emergency management team will be well-versed in the location or use of equipment that may be essential during an emergency. Consequently, the following tips will help provide guidance in writing this section of the plan:

• Identify critical equipment and control devices on maps. The facility diagram in the emergency plan should clearly mark the items such as shutoff valves for water, electricity, and gas; the telephone system demarkation; and the buildingwide HVAC (heating, ventilation, and air conditioning) controls. In addition, emergency personnel, such as fire and emergency response teams, will benefit from a list that documents a description or photograph of each of these items, its exact location, and any special tools needed to operate it. Maps should also identify caches of first aid supplies; emergency response kits; other essentials, such as fire extinguishers or bullhorns; and important paper documents, such as material safety data sheets.

• Mark the rooms. Because staff members often must react without the benefit of referencing the emergency plan, rooms that contain emergency supplies (such as crisis kits and first aid supplies) or important equipment should be clearly marked. The location within the room should be marked as well. For schools that do not have a telephone in every classroom, phone locations should be identified by placards or other insignias.

• Locate the equipment. Most staff will have few reasons to use emergency equipment and supplies during the course of a normal school year, so members of the emergency management team should tour the facility at least twice a year to locate the items detailed on facility diagrams. If practical, emergency response team members should also have an opportunity to handle and use (or simulate use of) specific pieces of equipment.

• Post instructions. Operating instructions should appear in the plan as well as at the site of the equipment or supplies. Although custodial staff may be well trained in shutting off utilities to the school, other emergency management team members may have little or no experience with these tasks. As discussed in Strategy 11, the language in the instructions should be straightforward.

Make Sure That It All Works and Is Present

Someone on the emergency response team, referred to as the "logistics and supply officer" or "plan monitor," should be responsible for verifying all emergency equipment is in working order and all supplies are present in a yearly audit. Although some of these tasks can be delegated, such as having the school nurse provide the first aid supplies, it is ultimately the responsibility of the logistics and supply officer to report that this emergency preparedness task has been completed.

CONCLUSION

Emergency preparedness is all about planning in advance, operating from worst-case scenarios, and delegating assignments so all involved have a sense of duty and responsibility. Fortunately, most school personnel will never really have to test their complete plans, but they will have a feeling of accomplishment and well-being that comes from being prepared. That feeling is just one of the many intangible aspects of an individual's job that makes it personally and professionally rewarding.

STRATEGY 13

Assessing Student Threats of Violence

A School's Response to a Growing Problem

With what seems like increasing frequency, school personnel are confronted with student-generated threats of violence toward people or property.

Unfortunately, some of the words that raise a red flag have now become part of the everyday language of many students, making it difficult to discriminate between the benign and the dangerous. The good news is many of the threats of violence that come to the attention of authorities do not indicate a real intent on the part of the student to carry out the act. The bad news, however, is that the threat is sometimes very real.

Fortunately, several organizations have studied the issue of student threats of violence and have released findings that will be helpful to those of us on the front line that must respond when an utterance, written document, or rumored threat surfaces. *The Final Report and Findings of the Safe Schools Initiative* and *Threat Assessment in Schools* were prepared by the U.S. Secret Service and the U.S. Department of Education (2002a, 2002b). These two resources include a number of specific response strategies for educators to use while investigating, evaluating, and managing threats of violence. Another noteworthy resource, *The School Shooter,* was published by the Federal Bureau of Investigation (1999). This document includes recommendations for a classification system for threats and an assessment model for use by those charged with evaluating a student threat of violence. Finally, *Early Warning, Timely Response,* published by the U.S. Department of Education (1998), offers general and specific strategies for intervening in and responding to threats of violence and to emergency and crisis events that can affect school safety.

USE THE RESEARCH AND A PROCESS

In the twenty-first-century classroom, teachers would be practicing antiquated methods of instruction if they did not use the most up-to-date information on brain-compatible learning, differentiated instruction, and the multitude of other research-based techniques for increasing student achievement. Likewise, school administrators should use the most up-to-date research related to analyzing and processing student threats of violence. This is one subject where school leaders need to be right every time.

The process is multilevel. The first level should include the following steps:

- An initial determination if the threat of violence is serious. Anyone who has worked in a school knows students periodically threaten to fight or engage in injurious behavior. Threats that by the nature of the language or wording reference the taking of life, serious debilitating injuries, or extreme property damage should be separated from threats of a lesser degree.

- If the threat of violence reaches the level of seriousness that one must ask, "Does the individual have the means and capability of carrying out the threat?" There is a difference between the threat to make a bomb and bring it to school when it is verbalized by a sixteen-year-old and when the same threat is made by a five-year-old.

- Is there any indication the student has taken steps toward following through with the threat? Using the previous illustration, a step taken toward making a bomb might be obtaining instructions, purchasing material to make a device, or even making an inquiry as to where those items could be obtained.

- Finally, is there any indication the threat is imminent? If so, what steps should be taken immediately to protect all students and staff?

The second level of the process is reserved for those threats that are deemed to be serious, have some level of credibility, and situations where school personnel believe further analysis is warranted. For these threats the best practice is to use a threat assessment team to dissect the threat itself and to analyze the student reportedly making the threat for a better understanding of each using the aforementioned research. Typically, a threat assessment team is composed of individuals having specialized training, expertise, or access to needed resources that will aid in the analysis. Members may include one or more of the following:

Administrative representative

Counselor

School nurse

Social worker

School resource officer or security personnel

Staff members having in-depth knowledge of the student making the threat

The charge of the threat assessment team is twofold.

1. Based on the analysis, what is the probability the student will carry out the threat? Is there any indication the student has taken overt steps and is engaged in planning? Although no planning has occurred, is the student adamant the threat will be carried out? Is there any history that indicates the student might be capable of violent behavior?

2. Based on the conclusions from the analysis of the threat and the individual making it, what course of action should be undertaken by the school? While the final decision at the school level will ultimately fall on the administrator, the team can and should participate in that discussion. Actions can be many, and may include the involvement of or referral to outside agencies; these actions can take place at any point in the process. For example, if the team obtains information that indicates the threat is much more imminent than originally thought, school leaders should be prepared to react quickly and decisively. If the team comes to believe the threat is not realistic, however, the student may only need to be dealt with from a discipline perspective.

Take a few minutes and conduct your own quick analysis of the scenario below, and consider how your staff might respond.

THE SCENARIO

It is Monday morning and the first bell has just sounded. The football coach tells you he overheard the players talking this morning during workouts about a fight that occurred Saturday night when some kids jumped "one of the weird kids who hangs out in the commons." The coach says the players heard a rumor the student who was jumped was going to bring a gun to school to settle things. The coach said that the students identified the student making the threat. The players told the coach the student "is a coward and wouldn't really do it."

You know the suspected student dresses in all black and is usually in the student commons area with other students of similar appearance. Although the student has not been a discipline problem in the past, there are ongoing academic failures evident.

Questions
- What action do you believe your staff would take if a similar conversation was heard?
- Would your staff simply find it unbelievable or think it was just one of many rumors heard in a typical school year?

- Might your staff do nothing because they would assume you already had similar information?
- Are there already pieces of information in the scenario that give you some guidance as to how to proceed?
- What might be your initial actions?
- At what point during your initial investigation would the threat assessment team be assembled?

Responding to student threats of violence is never easy, and no one wants to make the wrong decision in determining whether or not the threat is "real." It might be easier to always assume the worst and take actions based on that premise, but that is not fair to students and may create dissension within the school community. School personnel should develop a systematic response based on board policy, related educational research, and the need to provide a safe school environment for everyone.

STRATEGY 14

De-escalating a Situation With an Angry Parent

You'll Never Have to Answer for What You Don't Say

Understanding how to defuse the situation with an angry parent may prevent an argument from becoming violent.

Imagine you are at a Friday evening basketball game with your school's biggest rival. At the end of the game, your school has lost by one point. As the players leave the court, you observe the father of one of your school's players corner the coach and berate him, using profanity. The player's mother is attempting to convince the father to leave, but to no avail. The situation is quickly escalating, and the coach is looking for someone to intervene.

You know that

- this particular parent has been cautioned before about his behavior at school sporting events,
- there are other parents still in the gym, and
- the school principal is outside on the parking lot managing traffic flow.

Has this happened at your school? Unfortunately, it probably has. Whether in the gymnasium or the school office, principals and teachers are sometimes forced to deal with verbally aggressive adults.

Before reading further, take a few minutes to identify the key pieces of information that might determine how you could start to de-escalate the situation and consider the actions you would initiate.

WHAT TO DO

Although most conversations with parents are civil and productive, there will be times when communication about an unfortunate incident will result in the parent becoming verbally aggressive. Sometimes it occurs during a phone conversation, and sometimes it happens face to face. Either way, there are a few tips you will want to remember.

- Stay calm and listen. All parents have the right to be heard, and angry parents are no exception. Remember you will not be able to solve the real problem until all parties can communicate openly, honestly, and without malice. Think of the angry parent as a client, rather than as an adversary. This can put an emotional distance between the two of you that will enable you to treat the situation rationally and professionally.

• Do not take anything personally. Although an angry parent may say things of a personal nature, as an educator you must keep your remarks on a professional level. Some parents deserve the same type of "learner leeway" you give students. Remind yourself that angry people are experiencing many of the physiological signs of stress, including increased heart rate, difficulty listening, and tunnel vision. These physical changes make it exceedingly difficult to communicate with them, so choose your words accordingly.

• Use a low tone of voice. Appearing agitated or yelling back will serve little purpose other than to fuel the fire you are trying to put out. There are times when it is even advisable to speak so softly the parent must strain to understand what you are saying, which may serve as a distraction from the anger.

• Try to move to a more private setting. Separating an escalating, verbally aggressive person from an audience may remove part of the reason for the behavior. In most situations, however, it is not advisable to put yourself in a one-on-one setting with an angry person. If possible, have another school employee with you for the discussion.

• If possible, take notes with the individual's permission to do so. Whether the conversation is taking place on the telephone or in person, say, "I want to make sure I understand all of your concerns. Do you mind if I take some notes?" This sends two powerful messages: First, it indicates you want to remember exactly what is being said so you can resolve the issue—taking notes provides an accurate form of documentation. Second, it puts the parent on notice that his remarks are being recorded for further reference. This alone may cause some parents to eliminate foul language or threats from their part of the conversation.

• Do not interrupt. Interjecting "Yes, but . . ." to correct inaccurate statements may escalate, rather than de-escalate, the conversation. Even if the parent's statements are not based on the facts as you know them, it is usually counterproductive to try to insert your own perspective or to correct any inaccuracies at that time. Wait until the parent is finished and then diplomatically provide information from the school's perspective.

• Do not use such phrases as, "Calm down," "I understand," or "I know what you're going through." Parents may interpret these phrases as condescending or arrogant, even when they are not intended as such. In many instances, you will not be able to empathize or understand what the parent is experiencing, and to imply that you do may be considered patronizing.

• Ask for parental help in solving the problem. Jot down possible solutions from both the school's and the parent's perspective. After being heard, parents are often willing participants in a rational and productive problem-solving conversation.

• Assure the parents you are willing to listen carefully and to consider all possibilities. Although you may not be giving them the answers they want to hear, you can tell them that someone on staff will revisit the circumstances surrounding the problem to make certain the information is accurate. If the problem needs to be investigated further, provide a time frame to speak with them again. Giving daily or periodic updates on the investigation can help reassure parents and remind them of the school's genuine desire to be fair and consistent.

• Maintain eye contact without staring. Keep your hands at your sides and never touch or point at an agitated individual. If you are seated behind a desk, do not make any quick movements; this may further inflame the problem. If you are standing, maintain ample personal space between the aggressor and yourself. Moving into another person's body space when he is upset will not serve any positive purpose. If possible, stand at a ninety-degree angle from the approaching person. This may be less likely to be viewed as confrontational and might help defuse the situation. Keep in mind that different cultures perceive personal space in different ways; be sensitive to and take clues from the parent's body language.

• Take a few deep breaths and think before you speak. Even if the pause in the conversation is a bit uncomfortable, use caution and reflection before proceeding so the parent does not become angrier and more upset by your tone or choice of words. Remember, sometimes the best communicating you will do is with your ears.

THE SCENARIO REVISITED

In the scenario, initial actions should include diplomatically removing the parent or the coach from the scene of the confrontation. Because the parent's initial anger is directed toward the coach, redirecting his focus toward you may enable you to alter the environment in which the conversation will continue. It may be advantageous to say, "I want to hear your concerns, but let's get out of this crowd so we can talk," or to set an appointment for the parent to come in at a later time. This removes both the coach and the audience from the situation and allows for a cooling-off period.

Because the parent in our scenario has been warned before about his behavior, this confrontation may indicate he is not complying with established behavior. Summoning another staff member or security staff should provide added safety for all. From the facts in the scenario, you know the situation is escalating quickly and may require the removal of the parent.

In that case, it is always best to have additional school or law enforcement personnel present.

Although every situation will be different and individuals will not always react the way you hope, understanding best practices of how to interact with verbally aggressive people will give you a better chance of successfully returning to normalcy.

STRATEGY 15

Fights at School

Breaking Up Is Hard to Do

Prepare yourself and your staff members to deter fights in your school and handle them effectively when they occur.

When an administrator is alerted that there is a fight in the school, the news usually causes apprehension. The heart rate accelerates and adrenaline rushes through the body—and for good reason. Fighting is one student behavior that carries with it a significant probability someone will get hurt and the educational climate of the school will be negatively affected. On top of everything else, school staff will likely have to spend a great deal of time after the event sorting out the facts surrounding the altercation.

A DIFFICULT SITUATION

School personnel have both a legal and an ethical obligation to ensure the safety of all students. As a result, staff can find themselves in situations—such as witnessing a fight between two or more students—that, if not handled correctly, may result in victimization and injury. This is a particularly difficult situation at the secondary level because students often have the bodies and physical strength of adults, with the coping skills of adolescents.

One problem is most schools offer little if any staff training for verbal or physical de-escalation. Although colleges and universities provide instruction in classroom management, there is seldom any coursework related to managing aggressive individuals or violent incidents with multiple participants. Even when training is provided, it is often inadequate. Physical intervention methods are taught to school staff at walk-through speed, with compliant partners, and under little or no stress. There is little similarity between this training and what staff will encounter during an actual fight.

Another problem occurs because the dynamics of a fight create circumstances that work against those who try to intervene. The combatants in a fight will exhibit the physical and mental characteristics of stress, which are brought on by large amounts of adrenaline released in the body, and experience a reduction in sensory perceptions, such as the following: They will have little, if any, peripheral vision. The ability to process sounds around them will be significantly limited, which explains why they may not see or hear staff who try to intervene. Finally, combatants may continue to fight even when they are feeling pain.

Because of a lack of knowledge or a fear of "going on the record," some districts are hesitant to provide written guidance that instructs staff in how or when to intervene when a student fight erupts. The result is, staff does not know what is expected of them.

TAKE STEPS TO PREVENT FIGHTS

The student code of conduct should clearly communicate to students that fighting is prohibited on campus, and that there will be a disciplinary consequence for both the combatant and bystanders who encourage or instigate an altercation. Penalties for interfering with the ability of a staff member to get to or break up a fight should also be written into the student code of conduct and strictly enforced.

Sometimes the threat of a suspension for fighting has the least deterrent value in keeping students from engaging in this behavior. It will be what they have to do or are not able to participate in on returning to school after the suspension that may have the greatest effect on reducing their willingness to engage in a fight. For example, consequences could include participation in a support group for anger management, exclusion from activity programs, or community service. Some high schools train combatants to serve as peer mediators or require that they serve on a "jury" for another student accused of misbehavior on campus.

The teacher handbook should include directives for an appropriate response to a fight. Districtwide practices and procedures should be covered thoroughly, and this information should be included as part of the first faculty meeting of the year.

Supervision should always be planned strategically. This is especially true when considering preventive measures for deterring fights. Knowing when and where altercations are likely to occur on the basis of past occurrences should dictate where staff members are placed for supervisory duties. Adult presence is a strong deterrent to a number of disciplinary problems, and fighting is no exception.

HOW TO RESPOND EFFECTIVELY

The following advice should be kept in mind when preparing to intervene in a fight:

- Anticipate that assistance will be necessary and get other adults to the scene whenever possible. Remember, there will be a minimum of two combatants, and bystanders may also pose a problem. A single staff member will usually be ineffective and could even become a victim.

- On arriving at the scene of a fight, remain in control of your own emotions and assess the situation and surroundings. Remaining calm will help reduce the negative effects of stress mentioned earlier. If time allows, communicate with the other adults in the vicinity to determine who will disperse bystanders, who will interact with combatants, and so on.

- Remove the audience. Getting student leaders within the crowd to disperse is important because other bystanders will tend to follow. Removing the audience can eliminate a prime motivation for the fighters.

- Remain at least an arm's length away from those involved in the fight. (Although see the point below that begins, "Only as a last resort.") Instead, stand where there is a reasonable chance of making eye contact with one of the combatants.

- Identify the combatant with whom you have the most rapport and then give direct verbal instructions. Remember, everyone involved will experience selective hearing and vision. Clear, short, and concise sentences are more likely to be heard and understood. Use a firm, commanding voice to say something such as, "Daniel Jones, stop fighting now!" If a weapon is involved in the fight, law enforcement should be notified immediately. School personnel—with the exception of school police—seldom have the training necessary for disarming an armed student.

- If necessary, create a diversion to break the concentration and gain the attention of the students fighting. A loud, unexpected noise such as slamming a book to a wall or floor may interrupt and break concentration. Throwing water on the combatants has also been known to work. Once you have the attention of the participants, follow up quickly with succinct verbal commands.

- Only as a last resort should you attempt to physically intervene in a fight if you are the only adult present. You should do so only if you are able to help without becoming a victim, and only to prevent serious injury from occurring. If forced to do so, push and shove rather than grab, and then back off quickly. The shock of being pushed and shoved, along with the resulting loss of balance, may bring some reality back to one or both combatants. Remember that many staff assaults and injuries that occur during a fight are the result of getting between those engaged in the altercation.

- Once the combatants have been separated, immediately order or escort each student to an area where they cannot see or communicate with each other. In the immediate aftermath of a fight, it is common for both individuals to want to continue to "mouth off," and fights can resume as a result.

- In the aftermath of a fight, it is always a good idea to debrief the staff members who responded to the incident. This is an opportunity to discuss what worked and what did not. This information can then be shared at the next faculty meeting so staff can all learn from what a few experienced.

A proactive stance against fighting is always better than a reactive one, and the single most effective deterrent is visible adult presence throughout the school building. However, even under the best of circumstances most schools will still have a few altercations throughout the school year. When this happens, staff with training in how best to respond will have a better chance of intervening in a manner that successfully minimizes staff and student injury.

STRATEGY 16

Head 'Em Up! Move 'Em Out!

Relocating Students During an Emergency Event

Ensure that your school is prepared to relocate students during an emergency. Moving hundreds or thousands of students off campus with little or no warning is a daunting task, and it will be made even more difficult if advance preparation has not been thorough. While there may be an occasion when an evacuation is conducted with some advance warning, the greater chance will be that students and staff will need to vacate the school building in a short amount of time. Whether as a result of a gas leak, chemical spill, or sudden damage to the school building, the odds are that during the lifetime of an educator this type of event will occur at least once. When it does, planning will be critical.

Successful relocation—including the selection of the relocation site, having adequate supplies on arrival, and having well-thought-out student release procedures—affects the safety of students and staff members, and depends on the attention to detail during planning. Consequently, school leaders should consider the following:

• Choose more than one relocation site. When practical, identify at least three relocation sites. Two should be within walking distance of the school and in opposite directions from each other. This is important because the nature of the evacuation may determine the walking routes that are available or the event may render one of the relocation sites unsafe. The third site should be farther away from the school, to be utilized should the reason for the relocation affect a larger geographical area than that immediately surrounding the school.

• In the latter situation transportation issues become much more important. Therefore, planning should include school district transportation staff. It may be necessary to mobilize buses or other types of mass transit. In some situations, the school buses themselves may become temporary sheltering locations.

• Specify duties and responsibilities of the emergency response team. The school's emergency response plan should detail the relocation procedure, and specify duties and responsibilities of staff. Most plans, if properly worded, will already have a page of general duties and responsibilities that relate to a variety of emergency situations. Relocating students off campus, however, is one of several specific types of emergency responses that should have its own detailed listing of staff duties and responsibilities.

Staff members should also discuss and plan how relocation would occur during the lunch period, before school, or at a cocurricular activity. These types of situations present another set of difficulties to add to an already complicated procedure (see Resources).

• Practice, practice, practice. As problematic as it may seem, practicing an actual relocation of students is the best way to verify the plan's components. How to practice may vary according to each school's circumstances, but there will be some problems during an actual event that cannot be anticipated in advance, and practicing will minimize the number of problems and provide some level of reassurance to the school community that the plan will work. In addition to conducting an actual relocation of students, emergency response teams should participate in tabletop exercises that simulate some of the procedural aspects. Regardless of how the relocation is practiced, incorporating emergency responders into the process is important so that, in an actual event, each will have some familiarity with how others respond as part of the overall plan.

• Debrief the staff. It is important to debrief after any actual or simulated emergency event; this is especially true after a relocation drill. If outside emergency response agencies participated in the exercise, they should be included in the debriefing. As part of the debriefing activity, designate someone in the group as the record keeper. It is important to document comments related to concerns, problems, and ideas for improvement during this process. Although it is tempting to skip the debriefing component, especially after an actual emergency or crisis event, we do not advise doing so. Debriefing is just as important as planning.

• Place an emergency kit at each relocation site. Each relocation site should have emergency relocation supplies available for staff members and students. These supplies should include name tags or badges, clipboards and writing tablets, pens and permanent markers, flashlights and spare batteries, basic first aid supplies, and student release forms. The emergency relocation supplies kits should be checked prior to the start of each school year by the plan monitor or logistics officer to ensure each is adequately stocked. Items using batteries and other dated material should be refreshed as necessary.

• Include instructions for parent pick up, staff supervisory duties, restrooms, and so forth. The plan should include where students will be assigned, and detail supervisory and other staff duties at the relocation site. Other considerations include where parents will be staged and how students will be released to them; restroom facilities; and primary and alternative communication systems. Local law enforcement officials should know the relocation sites in advance, and discussions should occur as to the logistical issues that may affect both organizations.

• Be prepared to direct traffic in the absence of law enforcement personnel, and cross-train staff members. Where appropriate, staff members should have reflective vest and traffic-control aids in order to assist students across heavily traveled thoroughfares. Although the relocation plan may call for law enforcement to provide this function, depending on the urgency to relocate, staff members may find themselves acting temporarily in this role for at least the first few minutes of an event. Staff should be familiar with the plan to the extent that individuals can quickly assume others' roles. Seldom will everyone be where they are needed at the start of a relocation event.

• Inform parents of evacuation and relocation procedures. Publish the general relocation procedures in advance and make sure parents have access to vital parts of the plan. Although some people contend that publishing your procedures in advance creates added danger, the greater risk is the confusion and panic caused by not doing so. Providing your procedures and expectations for parents can be accomplished through parent newsletters, handbooks, websites, and so on. Not every parent will remember all expectations, but for those that do remember, communicating with them will contribute to a smoother process.

• Designate selected staff as parent liaisons. Utilizing parent liaisons to help calm and manage parents is a sound and advisable strategy. These individuals should be chosen on the basis of their de-escalation skills, longevity within the district, and ability to relate to and positively work with the parent community.

• Ensure that the relocation site is available at all times during the school day. Many schools use neighborhood churches; in some cases, the church may not be staffed at all times. Work in advance with the staff and management at the relocation site to define the parameters for use so each has a satisfactory comfort level with the procedures.

Even with the best of plans for relocating students, unforeseen problems will occur. With thoughtful planning and practice, however, another layer of safety will have been added to the school day.

STRATEGY 17

Student Searches

A Practical Application

Periodically, every school administrator will have to respond to parents' concerns or complaints about the treatment of their children. Although there are a number of topics that may cause parents to make inquiries—special education services, discipline, teachers' behavior, and cocurricular activities—the search of a student's person or belongings at school or at a school activity can be a hot button, potentially generating parental scrutiny.

Some complaints by parents will originate from not understanding the differences between a school's threshold for conducting a search and the conditions necessary for law enforcement officials to conduct searches. In other situations parents will simply believe a school search is not legally correct based on their perception of a student's right to privacy. The result in a few cases will be a judicial review of the facts and circumstances.

School employees should recognize that searching a student for contraband might create potential safety issues for staff as well as for the student. When in possession of something illegal or prohibited, adolescents may react irrationally or in a manner that puts those involved in the search at risk of injury. So how can school personnel ensure a search is conducted safely and legally? Fortunately, the following simple steps will help reinforce what to do in preparation for, during, and after student searches. These steps are not necessarily legal requirements, but they should be considered as a matter of practical application.

KNOW THE DISTRICT'S POLICY FOR CONDUCTING A STUDENT SEARCH

Knowledge of school district policy, in addition to applicable case law, is the first step in conducting a student search that will survive a review by the courts and other concerned individuals. During the course of a school year, many schools use administrative substitutes, such as lead teachers or school counselors, to perform duties in the principal's absence. However, principals should not assume these individuals are knowledgeable about conducting a search. Administrators should make sure that all individuals who could potentially be involved in searches review and understand related district policy.

Just as the courts may have conflicting views and opinions on the topic of school searches based on the specific set of circumstances, staff might read a policy and interpret it differently. Therefore, it is important ample discussion and professional development occur with all staff members who might be called on to participate in a student search.

Administrators should also review the following questions with those who are authorized to conduct searches:

• Have policy interpretation issues been discussed with these individuals?

• Have these individuals received training on how to conduct a physical search of a student and the student's belongings?

• Do these individuals understand the differences between probable cause and reasonable suspicion, and the elements needed to reach the threshold for a legal search within a school setting?

• Have staff members received training in how to appropriately and accurately document the search in a manner that will satisfy school board policy?

DO NOT RUSH THE PROCESS

Although the life of school personnel can be hectic, time should not be the driving factor in decisions about whether to conduct a student search or how the search will be administered. In most search situations, taking a few minutes for thoughtful reflection may be the difference between conducting a search correctly and conducting a search that may ultimately fall under scrutiny or review.

BASE THE DECISION TO SEARCH ON FACTS

In many cases that end up in judicial review or generate a parental inquiry there are questions about whether there were sufficient facts or evidence to support the search. Most school district policies on student searches include the phrase "reasonable suspicion," but few districts offer specific guidance about what that term means. Ask any ten administrators to explain the term, and chances are you will receive ten different responses. As part of the aforementioned training, staff should receive information on what the courts state constitutes reasonable suspicion for school personnel. However, as the circumstances unfold in a particular event, it will be important to compare what is known with what is required to meet the threshold. Prior to the search someone must ask, "Do we have reasonable suspicion and will it meet the test?"

USE PROPER PROCEDURES
AND BEST PRACTICES

Some school district search policies lack information on the practical application of conducting a search. The following procedural and best practices can make a student search safer and more productive:

1. From the time a decision to search a particular student is made, the student should not be left alone. A request to use a restroom by a student during an investigation may be a ruse to shed contraband. When one of the authors was a school principal, she once found marijuana in a vase on a bookshelf in an office at the school. It was later determined that a student suspected of drug possession had been left alone in that office prior to a search, and that the student used this opportunity to hide the contraband and avoid disciplinary consequences.

2. During the search, the student should not be allowed to place hands in clothing pockets, book bags, or other personal items. In addition to the possibility that this may present an opportunity to destroy or further conceal contraband, a student may panic and attempt to harm those in the room or themselves with something they have concealed. If contraband is located or suspected during a search, the student should not be the one to remove it.

3. When searching for a weapon or drugs, it is well advised to have additional staff members present in case the student panics or becomes aggressive. In situations where weapons or illegal drugs are the objects of the search, law enforcement or security personnel should be present. In any case, always adhere to the adage of safety in numbers.

4. Just prior to the search, the student should be asked, "Do you have anything on you or at school today that you should not have?" If the student has other prohibited items that could pose a safety issue, the administrator will have advance warning and can respond accordingly. Although the initial object of the search may be tobacco, a student might admit to having illegal drugs, a weapon, or other prohibited items if asked this question.

5. Document the search. All student searches should be documented, even when nothing is found. Many parental complaints occur when a search produces nothing illegal or prohibited by the code of student conduct. Parents will sometimes view the lack of finding anything during the search as a reason to believe the search was unwarranted. A

search that may appear to be routine at the time it was conducted might become an issue weeks or months later, so thorough documentation is recommended.

Documentation should consist of the following (see Resources):

- The facts used to support the search, including what constituted reasonable suspicion
- The conditions surrounding the search, such as where it was conducted, who witnessed the search, the name of the individual conducting the search, and what specifically was searched (e.g., back packs, purses, lockers, or cars)
- What, if anything, was found during the search?
- Any written or oral statements by the student
- If evidence was found, who took possession of it and where it is now located

The decision to conduct a student search should not be taken lightly or without careful thought. For a principal to do so invites a possible complaint from a parent, or possibly even future judicial review. Remember that the process of safely and legally searching a student begins long before the actual search. It must start with a solid foundation of professional development and staff training.

STRATEGY 18

Managing Electronic Devices

Sending the Right "Signals" to Parents and Students

When administrators create policies regarding student use of electronic devices, several issues should be considered.

Although technological advances over the past decade have been phenomenal and have had a dramatic and revolutionary effect on educational environments, not all changes have been positive. Most school administrators have struggled to manage the issue of students who possess or use electronic devices on campus. These devices include cell phones (with and without digital camera capabilities, and with and without text-messaging capabilities), personal digital assistants, or portable music devices.

Until recently, many school districts generally prohibited the possession of electronic devices by students, but, as many school principals know from experience, enforcing the policy was easier said than done. Consequently, some districts now take the position of only prohibiting the *use* of these electronic devices while the student is at school, rather than trying to regulate the mere possession of the item.

Because there are differing opinions on the proper policies and enforcement practices districts should adopt regarding the use of electronic devices, administrators should consider the following issues:

- Issue: Parents believe they and their children need access to each other by telephone during the school day. Fact: While it is true some parents may need to contact their children during the school day due to emergency circumstances, school personnel are usually more than willing to take the parent's message, get the student out of class, and provide the student the opportunity to speak with a parent by telephone. If the need for parental contact is not an emergency, parents could still call the student's cell phone and leave a message that can be retrieved after school hours.

- Issue: Electronic devices disrupt the school environment. Fact: This can be the case if strict adherence to policies is not reinforced consistently by all school personnel. However, it is possible to restrict and enforce policies on the use of these devices during the school day. Guidelines and rules can be established regarding when or where students may use these devices. Disruptions to the educational process are then more likely to be related to the lack of enforcement rather to a relaxed policy.

- Issue: Cell phones can disrupt or overwhelm cellular service during a school emergency. Fact: Except in extreme events affecting a large geographical area, cell phones used during a school emergency would probably have a minimal effect on overall cellular service. Because most students would be under staff supervision during an emergency event, staff members can and should restrict cell phone usage by students. In some situations, a student with a cell phone might be an asset if other communication options are limited or nonexistent.

- Issue: Allowing electronic devices at school increases theft in schools because the items are attractive to other students. Fact: Although some increase of theft may occur, there are no studies or data to suggest a significant increase in this type of school crime. Cell phones and portable music players have become relatively inexpensive and do not have nearly the monetary value that they once had.

- Issue: Using personal digital assistants, laptop computers, or cell phones to send text messages during class time will result in an increase of student plagiarism and cheating. Fact: Student plagiarism and cheating are nothing new. The best deterrent has been and always will be teacher supervision during class time and a strictly enforced student code of conduct. In addition, teachers can eliminate these devices during test-taking situations by insisting students clear their desks of all items other than writing devices and paper, and then alertly patrolling the classroom during the test.

REASONABLE AND PRUDENT

Although many districts may continue to prohibit the possession of certain electronic devices at school, many of the reasons that were once used to form policies now have little basis for support. When contemplating changing or enacting a practice or policy that regulates electronic devices in school, school personnel should take the following points into consideration:

- Using or displaying cell phones should be prohibited during the school day. Exceptions may be warranted when the use of the device by the student is to report an occurrence affecting the safety and security of students or staff or under other approved special circumstances.

- The advent of cell phones with camera capabilities has caused concerns about pictures taken in school locker rooms, restrooms, or other locations where there is an expectation of privacy. In those areas, cellular telephones should be prohibited and students should be instructed to leave the device in lockers, book bags, or purses. This policy should be stated clearly on signs posted outside restrooms and locker rooms. Unregulated use of any camera by adolescents in a school setting is an invitation for problems to develop.

- Violations of rules governing the use and possession of electronic devices should result in the future loss of such privileges, in addition to any disciplinary consequence that may be imposed.

- Rules and conditions for the use and possession of electronic devices should appear in the student handbook.

Many school administrators have taken the position that even though the current policy prohibiting electronic devices is "still on the books," enforcing the rule only takes place when students openly use a device. This type of selective enforcement may lead to complaints alleging discriminatory practices. Therefore, schools may wish to craft a policy that more clearly addresses the real issue with electronic devices, including the inappropriate use of electronic devices during the school day.

STRATEGY 19

Full-Court Press

A Media Management Plan

For most superintendents and principals, interacting with the media is probably on their list of the top ten most dreaded tasks. Not only do school administrators worry about what they will be asked, but they also worry after the fact about what was said and whether it will be reported in the context intended. When the topic of the interview is a tragic incident or a high-profile event gone awry, the level of stress and accountability becomes even greater.

So what should school personnel know about working with the media, and how can they practice and prepare for the inevitable? To answer these questions, let's take a look at an event that could occur in any school and see how one might prepare and respond.

THE SCENARIO

It is the end of a quiet day. Suddenly, the calm is broken by the sound of a fight that has started in a hallway by the boys' locker room. Nearing the scene, you hear someone yell that the school nurse is needed. When you arrive, you find the music teacher, a first-year teacher, on the floor, unconscious and bleeding from numerous cuts to the face and head. Two other teachers appear to be standing guard over a student sitting on the floor a short distance away, and several staff members are gathered around the injured teacher.

A staff member informs you there was a fight between two individuals—one current student and a nonstudent, a recent dropout. You observe the student, who is being guarded by school personnel, and are told that the nonstudent fled minutes earlier. It is further explained that as the first-year teacher tried to separate the two male combatants, he was pushed and fell into the nearby window, shattering the glass and cutting his head.

Just as the nurse arrives, the sounds of emergency vehicle sirens signal the arrival of local police and medical personnel.

Later that same afternoon, as required notifications are being made, you are informed the injured teacher is at the hospital and may have permanent damage to one eye, as well as other injuries that are less serious. The nonstudent involved in the fight has been arrested by the police, and the student is being detained at the local juvenile facility.

In most communities, this type of situation will draw some media attention, and the district's response to the related questions can have a significant impact, either positive or negative, on the community's perceptions of the school.

Before reading further, take a few minutes to reflect on how you might interact with the media concerning the incident.

POINTS TO CONSIDER

Now, after you have formed some strategies on how you might proceed, consider the following guidelines:

- Never hope the situation will merely go away. This is a wish that will probably not come true. If you do not take the lead in getting the truth and facts out to the public, others will disseminate their "truth," so you may be forced to deal with misconceptions and unnecessary negative fallout.

- If managed appropriately, the media can be a tremendous asset to help inform the public of the school's multifaceted response to difficult situations, and can be a conduit for disseminating accurate and positive information. However, if the school spokesperson is unprepared, the result may not be as positive. Try to stay focused on the message that needs to be conveyed and plan accordingly.

- Pay attention to feelings. Although facts are important, schools are about people. After a tragic event, the public will want to know that school personnel care about the human factor. When speaking publicly after a tragedy, avoid robotic answers. Be sure to convey condolences and empathy, without accepting or assigning responsibility for the events. This is usually a good way to begin and end a press release or interview with the media.

- Remember the value of a written news release or statement. Interacting with the media is stressful, even when it is a positive news story. When it is bad news, emotions and other factors may cause information to not sound as intended. Using a written statement or news release that precedes or supplements a press conference or interview can be beneficial. Although many districts will use central office staff to prepare news releases, there are times when other personnel should be actively involved. Words in a written statement should be chosen carefully. This is a time to be succinct and diplomatic.

- Keep the language simple. Avoid overly technical terms or organizational jargon. The language that school employees use with each other is one thing, but how we speak to the general public requires something different. When the public cannot understand what school staff says, they may leave with a negative perception of the event.

- Don't overexplain. There is value in keeping the answers and comments short and to the point. Readers and listeners tend to draw conclusions from the first part of what they see or hear. Long answers usually dilute what you are trying to convey. Staff should resist the urge to elaborate when it is not necessary to do so.

• Prepare for questions and issues. A team approach to difficult situations is essential in preparing to interact with the media. Bringing together all the key players that have information and knowledge of the incident can be invaluable in anticipating what the media and the public will view as the most critical issues. Failure to use a team approach will be evident in media reports.

ANTICIPATING QUESTIONS

So, if anticipating questions and issues is an important step in preparing to respond to the media, what types of questions might be anticipated from the scenario at the beginning of the article? Questions for consideration include the following, among many others:

- Why was the nonstudent in the building? Had the nonstudent been observed prior to the altercation?
- What was the disciplinary history of the assailant when attending school? Was the assailant violent and prone to these behaviors? Why is the nonstudent no longer attending school?
- What is the extent of the teacher's injuries?
- Who was present in the area when the assault occurred?
- How many adults are assigned to supervision during school dismissal?
- In light of the incident, do you believe the current level of supervision is adequate?
- Does school staff receive training to break up fights? What does the training involve?
- What types of security measures are employed at the school to keep these types of incidents from happening?
- Will security be enhanced as a result of the incident?

REVIEW AND COMPARE

Review your initial thoughts on how you would act in response to the media and the public. Did you find that the suggested strategies alter how you might respond? Using event scenarios to practice media management with a team will allow you to be more effective if a real-life event unfolds. Difficult situations that cause media scrutiny arise every day. They are inevitable. However, unfortunate incidents do not inevitably result in negative press. Even the most negative of situations can be used to provide the message to the public that, although bad things do happen occasionally, the school's responses are appropriate and considered.

3

Professional Development

STRATEGY 20

Is Your School Up to Speed on Safety?

Principals need to review and discuss school safety policies and procedures with all staff throughout the school year.

At the beginning of each school year, administrators across the country provide orientations, professional development opportunities, and assistance to new employees about the way "we do things around here." These procedures include recording student attendance, computerized record keeping, school improvement plans, master schedules, lunchroom routines, emergency information, and disciplinary referral procedures. Although all of these procedures are important, administrators should reserve ample time on their orientation agendas to discuss specific matters related to the safety of students and staff. It is equally important to involve the support staff because they will also have roles and responsibilities during an emergency or critical incident.

The following are some of the safety topics that should be reviewed and discussed with all staff:

• Supervision. Administrators know the importance of adequate supervision. They should stress that all staff members must work together to effectively monitor students and their activities. Staff should be reminded that the supervision of students is especially critical between classes, during lunch, and before and after school. It is also a good idea to discuss supervisory expectations for the chaperoning of dances, field trips, or other off-campus school or cocurricular activities. Because support staff members are an important part of every school's supervision plan, they should be included in the discussions. Taking the time to discuss the principal's expectations before a problem arises will often eliminate the need for later staff disciplinary actions.

• Emergency response plans. All new employees should receive a copy of the school's emergency response plan. Depending on the specific position of a support staff, a complete copy of the plan may not be necessary, but each staff member should still receive general information. For instance, a part-time custodian or food service employee might not need a complete copy of the plan. Rather, that staff member would need information from the plan related to specific job responsibilities. Furthermore, if the school uses a flip chart in addition to a more comprehensive plan, the components of the flip chart should also be reviewed. Remember, this process will be a new experience for first-year teachers, so additional time should be reserved for them to absorb the information.

• Relocation sites and evacuation procedures. Most emergency response plans include provisions for at least one relocation site in the event the school becomes uninhabitable during the school day. New employees need to be knowledgeable about these sites; they should review the procedures that would be used if relocation becomes necessary. Evacuation procedures should be explained—including evacuation procedures for times when students are at lunch or at assemblies. Unfortunately, school emergencies may occur early in the school year so it is important to make this information an important part of the orientation prior to the beginning of school. Waiting until later to provide this information is ill advised.

• In-place sheltering. All staff members should understand the procedures that are to be followed in the event the school has a need to shelter students in place. During an actual emergency, these procedures can be nerve-rattling—even for seasoned educators. Principals should emphasize staff may have to take the initiative under certain conditions when there is little or no communication from the administrative office.

• Access control. Although most schools currently limit access within the school during the day, all members of the staff should be informed of their responsibilities related to this important practice. All staff can help in this endeavor by informing school visitors and guests they are to enter using specific entry points and check in with the office immediately on arrival. In addition, all new employees need to receive instructions about how to safely and effectively approach individuals who have come on campus who have not followed building procedures (e.g., they are not wearing proper visitor badges). This should include instructions on the appropriate response if a visitor seems to be under the influence of a chemical substance or is visibly agitated.

• Substitute teacher instructions. Certificated staff members need to understand the administration's expectations for planning for substitute teachers. These instructions should include seating charts, attendance procedures, adequate emergency lesson plans, a list of students that might require more supervision or special attention, a list of students who the substitute can normally depend on for assistance, emergency flip charts, and procedures in the event of fire drills or actual emergencies (see Resources).

• Teacher handbook. The teacher handbook will contain a considerable amount of safety information. Although the expectation is that teachers will read the handbook, principals should not assume this. Therefore, the first faculty meeting should provide the opportunity to thoroughly discuss the safety information sections of the teacher handbook, which should outline the expectations for staff behavior. This will help both new and veteran teachers. The most important aspect of the handbook is that all teachers have a copy of the most up-to-date edition, sign for receipt of it, and are held accountable for the information in it.

• Legal expectations. The principal should provide a review of existing school safety and discipline policies, and inform all teachers about any new laws, court decisions, district policies, or practices that affect school safety. This discussion should include procedural information related to the reporting of possible child abuse of a student. In all fifty states, school personnel are mandated reporters; the principal should inform them and remind them of their legal responsibilities. Part of this discussion should be what it means for staff to act within their scope of employment.

• Communication devices. Because school districts generally purchase equipment and services on the basis of the lowest bid, it is sometimes not unusual for the intercom and telephone equipment to vary within a given district and even within a given campus. Consequently, principals should provide written information to staff about how to access intercom systems, telephones, or any other two-way communication devices available to them.

• Disciplinary statistics. At the beginning of each school year, staff should receive the prior year's disciplinary statistics, including the locations most prone to inappropriate behavior. This statistical information should be reviewed and then appropriately analyzed and used in making decisions.

• Disciplinary referral procedure. Most schools have procedural guidelines about referring a student to the administrator's office for matters related to school discipline. Administration should provide new teachers with the written procedures and any standardized forms used in the referral process. This discussion should also include dialogue about the nature of infractions that should be sent to the office for administrative intervention, as well as the types of infractions and how they should be managed within the classroom. The principal should provide parameters for what needs the attention of a school administrator as opposed to what types of disciplinary infractions should be managed by the classroom teacher.

ADDITIONAL CONSIDERATIONS

In addition to the aforementioned considerations, individual schools or districts may have other safety information procedures considered critical to new employee orientation. As all good teachers and principals know, teaching is not as simple as just telling. Consequently, it will be necessary for new employees to reassemble at midyear to review and discuss the same safety topics and procedures. And, just as important as for the orientation itself, principals should retain a copy of the agenda for documentation.

STRATEGY 21

What Teachers Must Know About Safety

Because decisions made by faculty and staff members reflect on the school community, safety training must be a priority for everyone.

THE SCENARIO

After a scheduled early morning fire drill, the school was finally settling into a normal school-day routine. Thirty minutes later, much to the dismay of everyone, the piercing noise of the fire alarm sounded again through the school. As teachers and students filed out of the school for the second time, administrators suspected the alarm had malfunctioned. After students and staff had remained outside for fifteen minutes, it was confirmed that a sensor had not completely reset from the first drill. It was a combination of good news and bad news: no fire had been found, but valuable class time had been lost.

The following morning the principal read a disturbing email from a parent whose child reported that during the second fire alarm on the previous day the student's class had not evacuated the building because the teacher was helping students review for a test that was to be administered later in the week and she did not want to be disrupted by yet another evacuation drill. The parent questioned the wisdom of such a decision and wanted to know the school practice in such situations.

The principal found it hard to believe that this incident could be true—that there was not some misunderstanding—but the veteran teacher reported to the office and verified that the email was accurate. The teacher explained she was certain it would be a false alarm because it was in such close proximity to the announced fire drill that had already taken place. In addition, the teacher indicated students were held only for a few minutes, until such time as they reached a natural breaking point in the lesson. The principal was astounded and upset.

Do you find this unbelievable? Do you think it could not happen at your school? In fact, a similar situation did occur in 2004 at a high school in Missouri, and it illustrates the need for teachers to know and understand safety policy and procedure, and how their actions or inactions can undermine a parent's confidence in school personnel.

GUIDED DECISION MAKING

Most principals have said, "If only 'so and so' had responded differently, this would have been much easier to handle," or "What was the staff member thinking when that decision was made?" These questions are not just a tendency to play Monday morning quarterback about previous events and decisions. To varying degrees, the reputation of a school depends on the ability of employees to make good, sound decisions and to respond appropriately during a critical incident or event. As leaders, principals are responsible for ensuring that staff members are properly trained and provided with the tools they need to do the job. It is important, therefore, that the training be all-encompassing and that it take into account the need for a reasonable response to a variety of situations that have the potential for negative outcomes. So what should be included in this type of staff development?

• Teachers must understand their personal and professional liability. Ask any group of educators about the contents of the *No Child Left Behind Act* and you will hear a resounding response that it is about academic achievement. What is often overlooked in the law is valuable information contained in Section 2366 outlining the liability protection that teachers have, provided they are "operating within their scope of employment." This protection is often taken for granted, but, according to the law, teachers who operate outside their scope of employment or who show a "flagrant indifference" for the welfare of their students may lose that personal liability protection. Those teachers also place added burden on the administrators who must handle the aftermath of an event gone awry. At least once a year, preferably at the beginning of the school year, a discussion of professional liability should take place in every school.

• Teachers must receive written administrative expectations. Although it is a teacher's responsibility to know the particular practices, procedures, and policies related to his or her job assignment in a school and district, it is the duty of the administrator to communicate this information, document that it has been communicated, and provide the resources where further information can be obtained. It is impossible to cover everything a teacher needs to know related to school safety at the first faculty meeting of the year, so it is essential to provide resources and printed material in addition to annual discussion and training.

• Teachers must be trained in appropriate responses to classroom and school emergencies. Although they are relatively rare, real classroom or school emergencies that have the potential for catastrophic results do occur. Usually such events happen with little time for teachers to process information using normal analytical thinking skills. Consequently, staff members instinctively will revert to the way they have been trained and to the planning that has taken place. Without such planning or training, indecision, inaction, or delay may result. Emergency drills, such as fire, adverse weather, and in-place sheltering, are examples of training and planning. As recommended by the U.S. Department of Education, administrators should use tabletop exercises to train all faculty and staff members. These exercises can occur during a faculty meeting or other staff development time and are an excellent training tool.

- Teachers must be participants in school safety. Some teachers believe school administrators are primarily responsible for the overall safety of students and staff. Although administrators are ultimately held accountable for all that happens at school, faculty and staff must also be willing participants in prevention and intervention. One of the best ways to initiate this type of accountability among staff members is to delegate individual classroom safety audits to the teachers who use a particular room on a regular basis. For each classroom, a checklist of safety features, strategies, equipment, and documents should be provided to teachers at the beginning of the school year (see Resources). The individuals who are assigned to teach in or use a particular room are responsible for verifying that all the listed items are present and, as appropriate, that they know how to use or operate the article on the list. Holding others accountable will pay big dividends because staff members will be better trained and prepared to respond to school emergencies and crises.

All faculty and staff should receive training that enables them to intervene and manage escalating behavior when an individual threatens violence or aggression. Basic skills can and should be taught to all faculty and staff members by those who have expertise in intervening when an individual becomes aggressive. In many instances, faculty and staff will have only one chance to choose the right strategy to defuse an escalating situation.

School safety comes down to creating and maintaining an appropriate plan of action and providing the staff development component to support it.

STRATEGY 22

Training Support Staff to Respond Appropriately

School safety relies on training for everyone, not just for the certificated staff.

For many school administrators, providing meaningful staff development to members of the support staff can be challenging. But a safe school environment—and a school administrator's professional reputation—are affected not only by the faculty's actions during a crisis, but also by the response of those in support roles. Regardless of the scenario, the buck will stop at the principal's desk. When any staff member is unprepared or misinformed, the results can have tragic consequences, and negatively affect how the principal is perceived by peers and the school community.

Take a moment to reflect on the daily interaction between students and support staff at your school. Bus drivers, food service employees, custodians, and secretaries all have frequent contact with students: The school bus driver is the first and last adult many students see each day. Students who participate in breakfast programs interact with food service employees at the beginning of the day, and even more students have contact with these employees during lunch. Throughout the day, students walk by custodians in the hallways, classrooms, or commons areas. Students who visit or pass through the school office area interact with secretarial staff.

THE SCENARIO

For many years, Billy has been teased and humiliated by other students. He is small, wears glasses, and dresses precociously. One morning, as he waits at the bus stop, he hears the usual comments: "Hey, four eyes," and "You look like a fag in those clothes."

Three boys grab his book bag and throw it around, playing keep-away. As the bus arrives at the bus stop, one of the boys dumps the contents of the bag. The bus driver notices the boys taunting Billy as he gathers his belonging and finds a seat on the bus.

When Billy arrives at school, he is visibly upset. As he passes a custodian, he kicks a trash cart, sending it rolling away. The custodian tries to get Billy's attention to ask him to retrieve the cart, but Billy unleashes a string of profanities and kicks a nearby locker, then heads down the hallway.

After Billy gets his breakfast tray, a food service worker notices Billy is eating alone again. He is red in the face, and appears agitated. Other classmates sitting nearby are paying little attention to him.

Just before the tardy bell rings, a secretary bumps into Billy in a crowded hallway. She says, "Sorry," and Billy replies, "No, you're not. No one is ever sorry. I'm sick of this place." The secretary is surprised by his demeanor. She does not know quite how to respond, so she does nothing and continues on her way.

Shortly after school begins, the principal is summoned urgently to an art classroom to help with a student who is violently out of control. On her arrival, she sees the teacher and students standing in the hallway. She looks inside the room to see Billy sitting in a corner with a carving knife, threatening to cut his own arm.

Was this crisis preventable? We believe it was, and that members of the support staff who witnessed Billy before the crisis erupted were key players in the tragic sequence of events. Had any one of them responded at any point, this story might have had a more positive ending.

PROFESSIONAL DEVELOPMENT

A number of strategies are appropriate for training support staff members.

• Emergency management plans. The success of a comprehensive emergency response plan hinges on the understanding of all staff members. Some support staff will have specific duties and responsibilities that should be outlined. During an emergency, assignments may be made on the basis of who is available or closest to the scene. Support staff may have to supervise students, answer phones, or locate and operate equipment they do not normally use. Therefore, they should have a complete copy of the emergency management plan, as well as such documents as the telephone tree and guidelines for utility shutoffs, building security, and supervision.

• Staff development. To the degree scheduling will allow, support staff members should be included in schoolwide staff development for school safety. Training in such topics as first aid, evacuation, in-place sheltering, and supervision will help prepare these staff for crises. In the scenario described, it would have been helpful for support staff to have been trained in de-escalating aggressive behavior and subsequent reporting procedures.

• Incident debriefing. Debriefing should occur after any crisis, and support staff should be included. Even if they were not directly involved in the incident, they can learn from what did and did not work, and they can make suggestions for improvements.

• Support staff handbook. Including building-level expectations for support staff in the staff handbook is an excellent way to provide all groups with identical information about appropriate responses and procedures for potential events and issues. As an alternative, you may want to create a support staff handbook that includes many of the same things as the faculty handbook. As with other staff, within a few days of receiving the handbook support staff should be required to sign, indicating they have read and understood it, and that they have had an opportunity to ask questions.

• Extensions of the classroom. Buses and other areas that fall under the direct control of support staff members are simply an extension of the classroom and should be treated as such. All applicable rules should be posted in the cafeteria, on buses, and in hallways and should be communicated verbally to all students and staff members. Principals should encourage lines of communication between the certificated staff and those serving in a support role so concerns about student behavior can be shared.

• Supervisory techniques and expectations. Support staff should be given directions and guidelines for supervising students in their respective areas: custodians in the hallways and the student commons, food service employees in the cafeteria, secretaries in the office and the hallways, and bus drivers on school buses.

• Campus communication. Always include support staff in internal communications related to safety and security. Support staff should know they are a part of the safety process. They can be members of any building committee that supports a safe learning environment for students and staff members.

• Job-related expertise. Work with districtwide department heads who manage support service functions in an effort to include site personnel in strategies that strengthen facility safety. In some cases, support staff will be the experts on safety issues and can present the information to certificated staff. It may not always be about teaching support staff members—sometimes support staff will be the ones with knowledge they can provide to others.

COOPERATION

Just like athletics, school security is a matter of teamwork, and everyone's safety is enhanced when all have been trained and had a chance to practice the play on the field. In the previous scenario, some players were missing from the game plan and, as a result, the school's defense suffered. Support staff members are essential to creating a positive school climate. Make it a practice to include them whenever school safety is discussed.

STRATEGY 23

Intimidation, Harassment, and Bullying

Fear Factors in the Twenty-First-Century School

Bullying is a common threat to students' physical and emotional safety, but it can be reduced.

THE SCENARIO

You are walking through the student commons area when you see Jeffrey attempting to move through the crowd. Several other students are repeatedly stepping in front of him, blocking his path. Jack "accidentally" bumps into Jeffrey and knocks his book bag to the ground. As Jeffrey tries to collect his belongings, others in the immediate area begin to laugh, snicker, and call him a fag.

You know Jeffrey is small for his age. Jack is physically larger than Jeffrey, and is known for his athletic ability.

Although you probably do not see this type of incident occurring every day, chances are good that something similar happens from time to time on your campus. When it does, what is an appropriate response?

STOP AND THINK

Before reading further, take a few minutes and ask yourself some questions: What would you do if you saw this occur? Which students need your immediate attention: the victim, the bully, or the bystanders? Do you think teachers or support staff should respond in different ways? What about the school nurse or principal's secretary?

At first glance, this situation may seem easy to resolve, but don't be fooled. Harassment and intimidation, which may include bullying, can be difficult to address. Some students are reluctant to report such incidents. When questioned, many male victims will deny the existence of a problem because they believe admitting to victimization is somehow a threat to their masculinity.

Although some elementary schools across the country have chosen to adopt formalized bullying prevention programs, many secondary schools have been reluctant to do so. The reasons for this are varied, but one factor is that many secondary teachers believe it will be one more requirement in an already hectic schedule of teaching, meetings, and professional development. Either way, the issue will remain a problem until the school community makes a concerted effort to eliminate it.

TEN STRATEGIES

Discussing bullying in the student code of conduct is a good first step, but it is not enough on its own. These ten strategies can help school leaders at any grade level address bullying behaviors.

1. Provide a definition of bullying. Some staff will have preconceived ideas of what bullying entails, but the problem is broader than they may think. There are three components to bullying. First, there is the intent to harm another, either physically or emotionally. This separates bullying from accidental remarks or actions. Second, there are intimidating behaviors repeated over time, as opposed to a single incident of negative actions. Third, there is an imbalance of power between the victim and the perpetrator. One individual or group of individuals is perceived (by self and others) to be superior to another because of financial, social, physical, athletic, or another type of power.

2. Share the district's policies and consequences for bullying with the staff. Although some principals believe staff is already conversant on this topic, it is a good idea to provide the various documents that explain duties, responsibilities, and administrative expectations related to prevention and intervention. If your state has legislation on this topic, it would be wise to share this information with staff.

3. Using staff and student input, develop a map of hot spots where bullying is most likely to occur. This map should be revised throughout the school year on the basis of discipline statistics and information from students, staff members, and parents. The principal should ensure that hot spots are constantly supervised: before school, after school, during lunch, between classes, and during cocurricular activities.

4. Advise staff to watch for evidence of cyberbullying. This form of harassment is defined as using the Internet or mobile electronic devices to send or display hurtful or intimidating content. Principals should remind staff that students are sometimes reluctant to report these incidents for fear that the electronic tools may be taken away by parents.

5. Provide a list of some of the signs that may indicate victimization to teaching and support staff members. Staff members need to know the

warning signs of victimization in order to provide an appropriate response.

- Unexplained bruises or cuts
- Torn clothing
- Nonspecific pain, headaches, abdominal pains
- Academic decline
- Loss of possessions or money
- Outbursts of temper
- Symptoms of anxiety
- Loss of appetite
- Suicidal thoughts
- Poor school attendance
- Social withdrawal
- Dropping out of school
- Combativeness
- Depression

6. Provide support groups for students new to the school setting. Students who have a transient school history are likely to be victimized. Although participation should be optional, support should be offered and involvement encouraged.

7. Remind staff that bullying may manifest itself in the form of "gay bashing." Not only does this behavior create a hostile environment, but it can also have serious legal repercussions. Words such as *gay, queer, fag*, and *faggot* should not be tolerated. Staff members are in a perfect position to help students understand the inappropriateness of this type of language.

8. Advise victims to respond appropriately. Such actions as avoiding the bully, staying around friends or adults, refraining from an emotional reaction, and reporting incidents are always good advice for students who are susceptible to victimization.

9. Encourage bystanders to befriend the victim. If a bystander is not comfortable with direct intervention, the least he or she should do is walk away and refrain from being a silent participant. If the bystander remains at the scene of the incident, he or she may be considered one of the perpetrators by the victim.

10. Post a code of conduct in all classrooms. After posting the code, a class discussion should be held to reinforce the school's expectations related to harassment and intimidation. A sample classroom code of conduct might be the following:

- We will not harass, tease, or embarrass others.
- We will try to help anyone who is being harassed, teased, or embarrassed.
- When we know someone is being bullied, we will tell a responsible adult.

THE SCENARIO REVISITED

Let's go back to the scenario and the questions.

The person who needs attention immediately is Jeffrey. His books were scattered and he has been embarrassed and humiliated. Staff should go to his assistance and help pick up the books. If the timing seems appropriate, ask him to accompany you to a private setting. If not, have the school counselor speak with him later in the day. Tell him you saw what happened and seek further information. He may or may not want to give the details, but school personnel should listen carefully to what he does and does not say.

The next individuals needing attention are the students who were harassing Jeffrey. Without creating a scene, make a mental note of who they are and direct them to the office or ask the principal to send a hall pass for them as quickly as possible. Speaking to these students individually is more likely to help them understand the negative effects of their behavior. If they remain in a group, they may continue to feel empowered, even if they are seated in an administrative office.

Next, make a mental note of the bystanders and provide pertinent information to a school counselor or administrator. If a teacher has the victim or the perpetrators as students in class, there might be a time for further discussion and personal conversation.

To change the culture of a school, the behavior of the adults must change first. The most effective antibullying initiatives are ongoing throughout the school year and are part of the discipline policies. Significantly reducing harassment and intimidation will require everyone's participation.

STRATEGY 24

Holiday Blues

Responding to Seasonally Despondent Students

For most schools, the holiday season is a time of bustling activity with school dances, food drives, holiday assemblies, and the conclusion of the first semester. And, while this should be a source of "good times" for both students and staff, it can be one of the most difficult times of the year in terms of school safety and security for those that work in an educational environment.

It is no secret the holiday season may not be a time when everyone is surrounded by loving family and friends. It is a difficult time for some people, who feel isolated, lonely, or despondent. It is during this time of year that people are inundated with images from the media of what the holiday season "should" be. It can be difficult for young people to sort out fact from fiction in terms of how ideal families are portrayed.

THE MONTH OF DECEMBER

For many schools, the month of December may show a significant increase in the number of student disciplinary referrals sent to the office for administrative action. These referrals may be for relatively minor classroom disruptions, but it is more likely that the increase will manifest itself with referrals for disrespect, insubordination, or defiance. Additionally, student fights or assaults may increase; left unchecked, these behavioral changes will cause a major disruption in the school's educational climate. Children show symptoms of depression in a variety of ways. Their depression may manifest itself by display of antisocial behaviors, spiking disciplinary referrals to the office.

While we are not suggesting that these referrals be handled without using the student code of conduct, we *are* suggesting that staff would be well advised to monitor the types of referrals written—especially during the months of November and December—to determine if there are underlying causes that might be best addressed by something other than removal from the classroom or suspension from school.

TYPES OF DEPRESSION

It is no secret many young people suffer from depression; causes include emotional and biological factors. Some may have experienced a significant loss or have serious behavioral problems. All may be at a higher risk for depression.

As with many diseases, the severity of depression will vary from person to person. When anyone is suffering from a major depressive disorder, the ability to function as a productive member of society may be limited. Conversely, when one suffers from a less severe depressive state, the ability to function day to day will be manageable. The result may be an individual who simply does not feel well much of the time. There are others who suffer from a third type of depression known as bipolar disorder. These individuals display severe mood swings. For some, the mood changes will be gradual; for others, mood changes will be rapid and dramatic, with little warning to those around them.

SYMPTOMS OF DEPRESSION

One of the challenges educators face in school is that many students may display mood changes—particularly at the middle school level—that have little if anything to do with a depressive disorder. These mood changes are simply products of the physiological and psychological maturation that young adults experience.

Children who are experiencing a depressive episode may exhibit the following warning signs:

- Persistent sadness
- Withdrawal from family or friends
- Increased irritability
- Changes in eating or sleeping habits
- Frequent physical complaints
- Decreased energy level
- Indecision, lack of concentration, or forgetfulness
- Feelings of worthlessness or excessive guilt
- Recurring thoughts of death or suicide

While not every student who exhibits one or two of these behaviors is depressed, students who exhibit several over an extended period of time might need help.

Student depression can be linked to the holiday season and may contribute significantly to the onset of suicidal thoughts or attempts. It is important to remember that a student who is considering self-destruction may have little regard for the personal safety of others.

HOW TO HELP

The following suggestions may help to lessen the impact of the negative side effects of the holiday season:

- Educate staff on the warning signs of student depression. Talk about this important issue at faculty meetings, and provide research-based articles for staff to read and discuss.

- Be vigilant when dealing with disruptive students, knowing that the behavioral issues may be a result of a more serious condition. While a disciplinary consequence may be in order, do not forget to keep the student's counselor informed so appropriate interventions related to mental health can be provided.

- When possible, be proactive in terms of individual and group counseling. Instruct your counselors to facilitate student support groups related to anger management, grief counseling, substance abuse, and so on. These groups should be ongoing during the school year, but they will be particularly beneficial during the holiday season.

- Remind students to secure all belongings while in the school building and to refrain from bringing unnecessary valuables such as large sums of money, personal electronic devices, and so on to school. This should help to eliminate some of the temptation for possible theft on the part of students with limited financial resources.

DON'T FORGET THE STAFF

Members of the school staff may also suffer from depression during the holiday season. Although the warning signs of depression may manifest themselves differently in adults, these individuals also feel despair and sadness, and may find it difficult to be productive. Some may have difficulty dealing with students who are antisocial or disruptive. As a result, patience may be in short supply.

BE KIND TO ADMINISTRATORS, TOO

Finally, administrators are given and readily accept the responsibilities and challenges of managing schools in the twenty-first century, and they may find it difficult to remember to take care of their own physical and mental health, particularly during the holidays when demands on their time are so great. Students and staff always expect the principal to be functioning on all cylinders, but doing so requires a conscious and strategic effort. In embracing commitments to the school community, principals must ensure they take care of themselves, too.

STRATEGY 25

Tabletop Exercises

The Ultimate Tool for School Safety Training

For many administrators, the task of providing meaningful and timely in-service training for classroom and school safety is difficult.

Staff development time is a scarce commodity in today's education environment. As a result, most in-service activities for faculty members center on academic issues, and rightfully so. Training for support staff members is concentrated on job responsibilities and duties—again, this is the way it should be. But during an emergency or crisis event, a lack of preparation may result in greater tragedy and a tarnished reputation for both the principal and the overall school community, so care should be taken and time allocated for training all staff members for the role of first responder.

Tabletop exercises are a valuable tool for preparing all school staff to respond appropriately to a variety of emergency events. This method of training can be integrated with the multitude of other staff development programs. Best of all, the exercises take very little time.

SO WHAT IS A TABLETOP EXERCISE?

A tabletop exercise is a written scenario containing a set of circumstances and facts that create the need for the participant to problem solve and make decisions that will bring the event to a conclusion with as few negative consequences as possible.

While under the stress of responding to an emergency, staff will make decisions on the basis of prior training and practice, real-life experiences, or simply the will to survive. In a true emergency, little—if any—problem solving will take place. In a school environment, it is difficult to simulate the stress that staff will face in a real emergency, but by practicing and training with problem-solving tabletop exercises, school personnel can establish a knowledge base that may provide them with necessary automatic responses when analytical thinking skills are compromised.

To understand how an exercise is written and facilitated, we provide a sample tabletop exercise, one used to train teachers to respond to a possible weapon in a classroom.

Although some exercises may appear quite simple at first, staff will quickly realize the complexities as they begin the problem-solving process.

THE SCENARIO

You are the classroom teacher, and it is midmorning in your second hour class. The class is working on an assignment, and you are grading papers. Carol, a student who sits near the back of the classroom, comes to your desk and quietly tells you Gary, who sits across the aisle from her, may have a gun in his book bag. Carol tells you that when Gary opened his bag a short time ago, she thought she saw something that looked like a gun stuck down inside a side pouch.

Additional facts: Gary has been in trouble with the juvenile authorities and recently ran away from home. Carol is usually a reliable student.

It will be the job of the facilitator to guide the participants through the three levels of problem solving discussed later in this article (i.e., considerations, options, and actions) and prevent staff members from jumping ahead to "actions" until a thorough discussion of considerations and options has been completed.

DEVELOPING TABLETOP EXERCISES

Written exercises should be constructed in such a manner as to be realistic, create issues, allow options, and facilitate training.

• Be realistic. Staff members must believe that the events could occur in their respective areas of responsibility.

• Create issues. The exercise must include facts or events that force staff members to make decisions. In the sample exercise, Carol reports to the teacher what she has seen, which creates an issue of what to do once the conversation with Carol is complete.

• Allow options. Although policies and procedures may govern some portions of the participant's final actions, overall the decisions must be generated by what is most likely to work given the complete set of circumstances and the personality of the staff member. Exercises should have a limited number of facts so as to encourage free thinking.

• Facilitate training. The manner in which the facilitator guides participants through the tabletop activity determines the level of learning and experience that staff members will receive. Facilitators should thoroughly explain the necessity for training on the given topic, the dynamics created by an emergency event, the physiological effects on responders, and the overall instructional objectives of the exercise.

• Because staff members should understand the process to be used as they work through the activity, a thorough explanation—including examples of the three components of considerations, options, and actions—should be provided.

- Considerations. This component encompasses the facts and circumstances from which the options are developed. For a consideration to be valid, the participant should be able to articulate why it would affect the forthcoming options. For the sample exercise, one valid consideration would be whether the event is unfolding at the beginning, middle, or end of the class period. If Carol is reporting her observations at the end of the class, the options available to the teacher are far more limited than if the teacher is receiving the information shortly after class has started. What other considerations would be essential for a participant to consider when developing options for the sample exercise?

- Options. Staff members should be encouraged to think in unconventional terms "outside the box," and to offer all viable options during the discussion. For the principal, who is often either the facilitator or an observer, this will provide insight into how individual staff members might respond in an actual emergency. The facilitator should never be critical of any option provided, but rather should ask participants to identify both the positive and negative outcomes that might result from a particular option. Any discussion with an individual staff member who appears to be advocating an unacceptable option should be held privately.

- Actions. Whether the exercise is worked with the entire staff, in small groups, or individually, participants should be asked to evaluate options and determine what courses of action should be initiated. The facilitator should reinforce that, in some situations, the first actions taken may be irreversible, so staff members should thoroughly evaluate their decisions. Some responses, though reasonable and logical, may still result in tragic consequences. For instance, in the sample exercise, if the teacher sends Carol to the office to summon help and Gary concludes Carol's exit is related to his weapon, he may react violently.

MAKING THE MOST OF IT

Tabletop exercises can be conducted with mixed audiences that include law enforcement, school administrators, faculty members, and support staff members. Each group can discuss and solve the exercise from its own perspective. While the sample exercise was written to train classroom teachers, a similar set of circumstances can be developed to generate a broader view of the event and to train a wider variety of staff members.

A tabletop exercise can have unlimited value because any change in fact or circumstance creates a new event with new or additional considerations, options, and actions. Staff and faculty will enjoy this type of training, learn about themselves and their abilities to respond during an emergency, and be better trained when an escalating situation requires action. For principals, school resource officers, and others charged with training staff related to school security, tabletop exercises are a win-win opportunity for staff development.

STRATEGY 26

There's No "Substitute" for Good Safety

In every occupation, there are times when employees are unavailable because of sickness, family emergency, or vacation. When this occurs and an alternate, or substitute, is needed, the public assumes, and rightly so, that the substitute employee will be equally qualified.

This assumption takes on added meaning when a substitute's responsibilities involve emergency services or include ensuring care and safety of others. For example, at thirty thousand feet, a passenger hopes a substitute pilot has all the qualifications and expertise that the regular pilot has to handle an in-flight emergency. A patient assumes a substitute physician is qualified to diagnose and treat an ailment. Therefore, it stands to reason the general public would believe and expect that when a regular classroom instructor is absent from school and a substitute teacher is in charge, the substitute is equally qualified not only to teach, but also to respond quickly and appropriately to ensure the safety of students during an emergency.

Day in and day out, substitute teachers report for duty in schools across the country. More times than not, they are ill-prepared for the types of safety and security problems that they may face. Substitutes come from a variety of backgrounds, and, depending on the state, many are in the classroom without the most basic of education classes, let alone certification in a specific curriculum area. In some school districts, substitute teachers receive no training on safety issues at the district level. It can be a recipe for disaster, or it can be a problem that you as an administrator can manage with thought and planning.

SUBSTITUTE FOLDERS

It is important to organize paperwork so substitute teachers can find it quickly if necessary. Teachers should create folders that contain pertinent information for substitutes who are assigned to their classrooms. Following a standard format for the folders will make finding information progressively easier for returning substitute teachers each time they work in the school. Principals should ensure that teachers have prepared their substitute folders properly by giving them a checklist of folder requirements. This checklist should be attached to the inside cover of the substitute folder and be completed when the folder is given to the school secretary. The following components should be part of the substitute folders (see Resources):

• School emergency response plan. Substitute teachers should receive a copy of the school's emergency response plan or be made aware of where one can be found, and provided an opportunity to read it. In either case, substitute teachers should know the most important components of the plan. If emergency response flip charts are used in the school, the substitute should receive the flip chart as part of the substitute teacher folder. The chart will provide the substitute with explicit instructions of what to do under specific types of emergency situations. In addition, substitute teachers should receive individualized evacuation and sheltering plans for any students with special needs.

• Severe weather, fire evacuation, in-place sheltering, and earthquake instructions. The folder should also include information related to building procedures for severe weather, fire evacuation, and in-place sheltering, and what to do in the event of an earthquake. If procedures are posted in the classroom, the folder should note where procedures are located.

• List of student health concerns. Each school year, the school nurse should provide a list of students with specific health-related problems to all certified staff members. Because a variety of emergency situations can arise on any given school day, a copy of this list should be included in the substitute folder. This list should include the names of students who have such conditions as epilepsy, diabetes, and life-threatening allergies, and what the teacher should do in those emergencies. This folder should also include guidelines for sending students to the school nurse for day-to-day health events.

• Student disciplinary referrals. Substitute teachers should receive information about the proper procedures for referring students to the office for disciplinary purposes as well as the applicable building level forms. They should also be reminded that parents may have the opportunity to read the referral forms; substitutes should be encouraged to describe the student behavior only, and to refrain from using language that could be considered emotional or unprofessional.

• Seating charts. No one should ever expect a substitute teacher to try to manage—let alone teach—students without having a seating chart. Students simply cannot be allowed to sit at a location of their choice without teacher guidance and input, and the substitute is in no position to provide this type of information. Teachers should be required to have a classroom seating chart in the folders. When possible, the seating chart should contain pictures of students, as well as names. This can be accomplished relatively easily if the school uses picture identification badges for students.

• Emergency lesson plans. Teaching from bell to bell will keep students on task and minimize the time that they can engage in inappropriate behavior. Occasionally, teachers are faced with unexpected situations in which they do not have time to prepare complete and detailed lesson plans for the day they will be absent. Therefore, all teachers should be required to leave emergency lesson plans that anyone—regardless of certification—could teach.

ADDITIONAL SUPPORTS

Handbooks

Substitute teachers should be given—and required to read—a copy of the student handbook and the teacher handbook before or when reporting to their first assignment for the school year. There is no other document that contains as much information as the student handbook in terms of rules and regulations related to behavioral expectations.

The teacher handbook can provide a wealth of information about specific procedures, such as attendance procedures, school arrival information, classroom management expectations, and assembly guidelines. When a substitute teacher has had a chance to work within a building over a period of time, these procedures become second nature. For those who are relatively new to a particular school, however, this type of information can be necessary for success.

Critical Equipment

Locations in a classroom that contain emergency response supplies or equipment should be clearly identified. Although this safe school strategy should be standard in every school and classroom, it takes on added importance when substitute teachers are called on to respond in an emergency. Cabinets or drawers that contain first aid supplies should be marked. The location of the emergency gas shutoff in a science lab should also be clearly identified. Fire blankets, fire extinguishers, material safety data sheets (MSDS), and the like should all be easily located. A written list should be included in the substitute's folder for classrooms with this type of emergency equipment and supplies.

Buddy Up

Every substitute teacher should have a "buddy" teacher to turn to should something go awry and immediate assistance be needed. All regular classroom teachers who teach in classrooms adjacent to a class taught by a substitute should be instructed, as practical, to check on the substitute at least once a day to see whether any assistance is needed. In addition, regular teachers should make personal contact and introduce themselves as a matter of courtesy and as part of planning for safety and security.

CONCLUSION

As with most policies, practices, or procedures related to safety and security, the key to ensuring that substitute teachers can protect the well-being of their students is planning. No one expects regular teachers to be present in their classrooms every single day during the school year. But administrators, students, and parents can—and should—expect that teachers will prepare for their eventual absence. Substitute folders, handbooks, clearly marked critical equipment, and personal contact can give substitute teachers the support they need to do their jobs and maintain a high level of safety and security for their students.

4

Top Ten

STRATEGY 27

School Safety's Top Ten

The Top Ten Things to Remember
When Creating a Safe School Environment

School personnel understand that safety seldom comes down to any one particular component or plan, but rather that it is a combination of strategies and ideas that make a school safe and secure for everyone. As school employees and authors on the topic of school safety, the authors understand all too well that most school administrators do a great deal of reading "on the run." In keeping with this philosophy, we have created a "top ten" list of strategies that we consider essential to assessing the totality of the school environment as related to safety and security. Whether you read it on the run or take your time to read it carefully, we believe you will find a few new ideas to consider. You might also find information that will reinforce the necessity of doing some of the things you routinely do each school year.

10. PROVIDE STUDENTS WITH AN ANONYMOUS TIP LINE

Many states have a toll-free anonymous tip line that students, and in some cases adults, can use when they have information related to a situation that might be of danger to themselves or others. If your state has such a toll-free number, be sure to publicize it by posting the number in every classroom, and strategically throughout the entire building. The toll-free number should also be included in the student handbook. If students in your district wear or carry picture identification badges, the phone number can be printed on the badge. If your state or district does not provide a toll-free number for such use, we recommend developing other in-house methods for anonymous reporting, such as school answering machines with a designated phone line. But again, remember this will be of little value if students are not taught and reminded throughout the school year this resource is available to them.

9. DO NOT ASSUME THE DISTRICT'S MAINTENANCE DEPARTMENT OR OTHER OUTSIDE STAFF MEMBERS WILL MONITOR THE SCHOOL FOR SAFETY DEFICIENCIES

As the recognized leaders of the school, the principal and assistant principals have the responsibility to develop strategies that identify and remedy general safety issues. One of the best strategies available is the use of a safety team. This team should include the school nurse, a school counselor, support staff members, school resource officers, security personnel, and other certificated staff members. The safety team should periodically review school data, including accident reports, and conduct general inspections of the facility. Because no one person is an expert in all areas of school safety, the use of a team brings together a number of individuals with expertise in varied, specific areas.

8. DO NOT ASSUME PARENTS BELIEVE THE SCHOOL HAS DONE EVERYTHING POSSIBLE TO CREATE A SAFE CAMPUS

Most parents want to believe that school is safe. The media can have a significant influence on their attitudes, however, and the general public is routinely exposed to negative stories related to schools and school safety. Although parents may not ask you to explain the safety strategies you employ, do not doubt for a moment that they will want to know what you are doing. For these reasons it is important for staff to take the time to use the tools at their disposal to inform parents about the safety strategies the school employs. School websites, student orientations, handbooks, and newsletters are some of the avenues administrators can use to help keep parents informed about the school's safety strategies.

7. PERIODICALLY REVIEW THE SCHOOL'S EMERGENCY RESPONSE PLAN WITH ALL STAFF MEMBERS THROUGHOUT THE SCHOOL YEAR AND TRAIN WITH TABLETOP EXERCISES

It is not sufficient to discuss the emergency response plan at the beginning of the school year and then automatically expect faculty and staff to respond correctly during a critical incident. In an actual emergency, faculty and staff members will experience a high degree of stress, and their ability to rationally problem solve may be significantly impaired. Therefore, we recommend that school personnel periodically be given the opportunity to practice and train for emergency situations through the use of tabletop exercises. These exercises can cover such topics as emergency events that might occur at cocurricular activities, or they might simulate such events as a weapon in the school or a student or staff member death that occurs during the school day.

6. DO NOT ASSUME STUDENTS WILL AUTOMATICALLY COME FORWARD WITH CRITICAL SCHOOL SAFETY INFORMATION BECAUSE IT IS THE RIGHT THING TO DO

Students have to be educated throughout the school year on the topic of safety, and teachers should be required to teach the student handbook with a particular emphasis on the sections pertaining to student reporting. We also recommend the use of tabletop exercises written specifically for students. These exercises can easily be included in health and physical education classes, or in homeroom and student advisory activities.

The tabletop exercises should include discussions of real-life scenarios where students evaluate pieces of information involving safety and then determine the proper course of action. The result will be students who are better prepared to think critically and rationally during a school or personal emergency.

5. HAVE A VARIETY OF INDIVIDUALS REVIEW THE EMERGENCY RESPONSE PLAN EACH SCHOOL YEAR

Although superintendents and principals have a great deal of expertise related to school safety, no one individual can anticipate and understand every facet of a school environment. It is therefore imperative for other school personnel—such as school nurses, custodians, secretaries, teachers, counselors, school resource officers, and other administrative personnel—to read the emergency response plan carefully and be allowed to suggest additions and deletions as deemed appropriate.

Principals should never let their egos get in the way of emergency planning and management. Each crisis and emergency drill should have time allotted for debriefing. For routine drills, such as severe weather or fire evacuations, this debriefing can be as simple as sending an email to staff members asking for their personal evaluations of how things went and if they have any suggestions for improvement. For other drills, such as in-place sheltering or relocation drills, the emergency response team should assemble after the event but on the day of the drill, and discuss the event as a group. These meetings should be documented and any recommendations shared with the entire staff.

4. DO NOT ASSUME LOCAL EMERGENCY SERVICE PROVIDERS WILL BE ABLE TO PROVIDE IMMEDIATE ASSISTANCE DURING A SCHOOL CRISIS OR EMERGENCY

In a crisis, depending on the location of the school, many staff members may find it necessary to "go it alone" for several minutes or longer until help from outside agencies arrives. In addition, the principal may have to manage the event without assistance from outside sources for quite some time. We suggest planning for a worst-case scenario that assumes staff members will have to handle some of the tasks that would normally be provided by responding agencies.

Staff members should be prepared to direct traffic if it becomes necessary to move students away from the school during an evacuation. Brightly colored vests should be located in designated crisis-supply kits and teachers should be trained as to their appropriate use. Sufficient first aid supplies for large numbers of injuries should also be available for staff and students. Staff members should be cross-trained to perform essential tasks. Students should also know where to access first aid supplies in the event a classroom teacher is injured during an emergency.

3. DO NOT ASSUME AN ADMINISTRATOR WILL BE PRESENT OR IN CHARGE DURING AN EMERGENCY

Principals are absent periodically throughout the school year because of meetings, conferences, and a variety of other duties that take them off campus for all or part of a school day. Make certain others on staff are prepared to take control when necessary. The ability of others to respond and lead appropriately will be a direct reflection on the planning and preparation a principal has made for a school emergency.

When conducting emergency drills or facilitating tabletop exercises, periodically place alternates in positions of command. Designated alternates within the plan will need the same amount of training as the designee, so make their training a priority.

2. STRESS THE IMPORTANCE OF DOCUMENTATION AND ENSURE THAT ALL STAFF MEMBERS DOCUMENT ISSUES AND ACTIONS RELATED TO SCHOOL SAFETY

A school employee's personal and professional accountability has never been higher than it is in the beginning of the twenty-first century. It is imperative that written records be kept for all staff training, drills, and event debriefings. This documentation can be in the form of faculty meeting agendas, in-service handouts, memos, emails, and written minutes of meetings related to safety and security. Like most safety issues, it is not a problem until it is a problem—and then it is a major problem. Consequently, keeping a written record of what has been provided to staff in terms of suggestions or mandates is very important.

1. AND THE NUMBER ONE SUGGESTION: DO NOT UNDERESTIMATE THE VALUE OF STRATEGIC SUPERVISION

Although technological tools and advances have a place in today's school environment, adult supervision is still the foundation of any safe school plan, and strategic supervision will have a positive impact on school safety. Considering the limited human resources available during the school day, knowing where and when adults should supervise is of extreme importance. Supervisory assignments should be based on the number of personnel available, a review of previous disciplinary statistics, anecdotal information from staff and students, and the type of activity to be monitored. It is not enough to make a general supervisory assignment to staff members; administrators should use strategic supervision to consider and recognize where problems are most likely to occur and assign staff members accordingly.

Resources

General Classroom Safety Checklist

_____ Classroom has room number or usage displayed and easily read.

_____ Classroom door lock works.

_____ Classroom door can be locked without stepping into hallway.

_____ Classroom door glass has cover present or available.

_____ Classroom windows have blinds or other type of covering.

_____ Classroom window locks function.

_____ Room lights are in working order with good illumination.

_____ Telephone or intercom access is at or near teacher's desk.

_____ Phone directory is current and easily accessed.

_____ Emergency telephone numbers are readily accessible to all.

_____ Telephone usage instructions are posted.

_____ Violence hotline or similar type telephone number are posted.

_____ First aid kit or supplies are stocked and location identified.

_____ Severe weather and sheltering maps are posted (with primary and secondary locations).

_____ Evacuation and sheltering locations have been discussed with students.

_____ Flip chart is posted and reviewed with students.

_____ Laminated cards with room numbers for emergencies are easily located and accessible.

_____ Classroom rules are posted and discussed with students.

_____ The nearest fire extinguisher is located and more than one person is knowledgeable in its use.

_____ Free-standing bookcases and cabinets more than five feet tall are secured to the wall.

_____ Television is strapped or secured to a wall mount or portable stand.

_____ The room is free of trip hazards.

Emergency Management Team Duties and Responsibilities

Relocation Event

(Title in bold indicates recommended terminology by the U.S. Department of Education and the United States Department of Homeland Security.)

Positions	Person Assigned	Duties/Responsibilities
Team Leader: **School Commander**	Principal Alternate 1 Alternate 2	✓ Evaluate incoming information ✓ Determine emergency services needs ✓ Activate emergency plan and team ✓ Order relocation ✓ Request additional district services ✓ School spokesperson ✓ Precontact relocation sites ✓ Coordinate supervision of students
Communications: **Liaison to Emergency Providers**	Designee Alternate 1 Alternate 2	✓ Make critical calls (911) ✓ Take student schedules and/or class list to site ✓ Use emergency warning systems ✓ Oversee use of intercom system ✓ Notify band, choir, P.E., etc. ✓ Manage phones at relocation site ✓ Assist with student release ✓ Maintain event log
Medical: **Medical Staff**	Designee Alternate 1 Alternate 2	✓ Triage multiple victims ✓ Administer immediate first aid ✓ Determine need for additional care ✓ Direct immediate movement of injured from school site ✓ Identity tag on victims transported
Media: **Public Information Officer**	Designee Alternate 1 Alternate 2	✓ Work with district P.I.O. as needed ✓ Prepare for media contacts off site ✓ Assimilate information for CMT leader ✓ Assist student supervision ✓ Notify appropriate district officials as directed
Security: **Safety Officers**	Designee Alternate 1	✓ Secure bldg. if time allows ✓ Coordinate final bldg. searches

(Continued)

(Continued)

Positions	Person Assigned	Duties/Responsibilities
	Alternate 2	✓ Coordinate traffic control ✓ Interface with emergency service agencies
Staff Liaison: **Operations**	Designee Alternate 1 Alternate 2	✓ Assist with staff inquiries and needs ✓ Adjust student supervision assignments ✓ Keep team leader informed ✓ Assist with communication functions
Parent Liaison: **Operations**	Designee Alternate 1 Alternate 2	✓ Handle parent inquiries and contacts ✓ Assist with student transition during relocation ✓ Assist with communication function ✓ Assist with student release from relocation site
Plan Monitor: **Logistics**	Designee Alternate 1 Alternate 2	✓ Directly assist team leader ✓ Ensure adequate communication devices available ✓ Coordinate media function with team leader
Counselors: **Student Caregivers**	Designee Alternate 1 Alternate 2	✓ Assess students' emotional needs ✓ Gather data on injured or missing students ✓ Assess staff members' emotional needs ✓ Assist with parent inquiries ✓ Assist with student release ✓ Assist with student transition during relocation
Family Reunification (Double-gated system)	Designee Designee Alternate 1 Alternate 2 Use parent liaisons, communication and plan monitors to assist	✓ Set up double-gated student release ✓ Two staff per table to provide checkout form ✓ Two staff per table to greet parents and explain procedure ✓ Two staff per table to serve as runners to get students

Out-of-District Travel Safety Checklist

Event: _____

Staff Member in Charge: _____

Dates of Travel _____ # of Students _____

   ☐ Permission slips completed

   ☐ Emergency contact list and numbers

   ☐ Itinerary provided to students, parents, and school

   ☐ Pertinent maps

   ☐ Student medical and prescription information

   ☐ Expectation of conduct provided to students

   ☐ Chaperone instructions distributed

   ☐ Supervision plans

   ☐ Student statement forms

   ☐ Student and teacher handbook

   ☐ First aid supplies

   ☐ Accident or injury forms and procedures

   ☐ Camera

   ☐ Student belongings inspected

Student Search Form

This form can be used to document basic information related to the search of a student and/or personal items.

1. Name, gender, and age of student

_____   _____   _____   _____
Name   Gender   Grade   Age

2. School, date, time, and location of search

_____   _____   _____   _____
School   Date   Time   Location of search

3. Names, titles or positions, and contact numbers for officials authorizing, conducting, and witnessing the search

_____   _____
Official authorizing search   Title/position   Contact #

_____   _____
Official conducting search   Title/position   Contact #

_____   _____
Official conducting search   Title/position   Contact #

_____   _____
Official witnessing search   Title/position   Contact #

4. Statement of facts

Provide information supporting reasonable suspicion or other justification for search.

_____

_____

_____

_____

_____

_____

5. Details of search

Provide information on how the search was conducted, what (if anything) was found, admissions or statements made by the student, special or unusual circumstances, and other pertinent facts.

_____

_____

_____

_____

_____

_____

Substitute Teacher: Critical Information Checklist

Room # _____ Teacher Name_____

☐ Emergency response flip chart

☐ Evacuation and sheltering instructions

☐ First aid supplies

☐ Emergency backpack with supplies

☐ Map of school with legend

☐ Fire extinguisher

☐ Intercom and phone usage instructions

☐ Seating chart

☐ Student conflict issues

☐ Health and medical alerts

☐ Discipline referral forms

☐ Teacher handbook

☐ Student handbook

☐ Lesson plan

☐ Buddy teacher

☐ Alternate buddy teacher

☐ Special instructions

Bibliography

American Psychiatric Association. (2000). *Quick Reference to the Diagnostic Criteria from DSM-IV-TR.* Washington, DC: Author.

Barton, E. (2006). *A Bullying Prevention: Tips and Strategies for School Leaders and Classroom Teachers.* Thousand Oaks, CA: Corwin Press.

Beane, A. L. (1999). *Bully-Free Classroom.* Minneapolis, MN: Free Spirit Publishing.

Beaudoin, M.-N., & Taylor, M. (2004). *Breaking the Culture of Bullying and Disrespect Grades K–8.* Thousand Oaks, CA: Corwin Press.

Brunner, J. M., & Lewis, D. K. (2001). *Problem-Solving Exercises: Elementary Edition.* Springfield, MO: Edu-Safe Publishing.

Brunner, J. M., & Lewis, D. K. (2001). *Problem-Solving Exercises: School Resource Officer Edition.* Springfield, MO: Edu-Safe Publishing.

Brunner, J. M., & Lewis, D. K. (2001). *Problem-Solving Exercises: Secondary Edition.* Springfield, MO: Edu-Safe Publishing.

Brunner, J. M., & Lewis, D. K. (2001). *Problem-Solving Exercises: Student Edition.* Springfield, MO: Edu-Safe Publishing.

Brunner, J. M., & Lewis, D. K. (2002). *Problem-Solving Exercises: Support Staff Edition.* Springfield, MO: Edu-Safe Publishing.

Brunner, J. M., & Lewis, D. K. (2004). *Providing Teachers the Tools for Safe Classrooms.* Springfield, MO: Edu-Safe Publishing.

Brunner, J. M., & Lewis, D. K. (2005). *School House Bullies: Preventive Practices for Professional Educators.* Thousand Oaks, CA: Corwin Press.

Brunner, J. M., & Lewis, D. K. (2006). *Student Searches: A Practical Application for School Administrators.* Springfield, MO: Edu-Safe Publishing.

Federal Bureau of Investigation (FBI). (1999). *The School Shooter: A Threat Assessment Perspective.* Washington, DC: Author.

Federal Emergency Management Administration (FEMA). (2004). *National Incident Management System (NIMS), An Introduction Self Study Guide.* Washington, DC: Author.

Harris, S., & Petrie, G. E. (2003). *Bullying the Bullies, the Victims, the Bystanders.* Lanham, MD: Scarecrow Press, Inc.

Jaksec, C. (2007). *Toward Successful School Crisis Intervention Nine Key Issues.* Thousand Oaks, CA: Corwin Press.

Lee, C. (2004). *Preventing Bullying in Schools.* Thousand Oaks, CA: Corwin Press.

McGrath, M. J. (2006). *School Bullying: Tools for Avoiding Harm and Liability.* Thousand Oaks, CA: Corwin Press.

Moore, M., & Minton, S. J. (2004). *Dealing With Bullying in Schools: A Training Manual for Teachers, Parents and Other Professionals.* Thousand Oaks, CA: Corwin Press.

National Association of Secondary School Principals (NASSP). (2004). *Breaking Ranks II: Strategies for Leading High School Reform.* Reston, VA: Author.

National Association of Secondary School Principals (NASSP). (2006). *Breaking Ranks in the Middle: Strategies for Leading Middle Level Reform.* Reston, VA: Author.

Office of Safe and Drug Free Schools and U.S. Department of Education. (2003). *Practical Information on Crisis Planning: A Guide for Schools and Communities.* Washington, DC: Author.

Rigby, K. (2001). *Stop the Bullying: A Handbook for Teachers.* Markham, Ontario: Pembroke Publishers.

Roberts, W. B. Jr. (2006). *Bullying From Both Sides: Strategic Interventions for Working with Bullies and Victims.* Thousand Oaks, CA: Corwin Press.

Sizer, T. R. (1999, September). No two are quite alike. *Educational Leadership, 57,* 1, 6–11.

Smith, S. T. (2003). *Surviving Aggressive People: Practical Violence Prevention Skills for the Workplace and the Street.* Boulder, CO: First Sentient Publications.

Sullivan, K., Cleary, M., & Sullivan, G. (2004). *Bullying in Secondary Schools: What It Looks Like and How to Manage It.* Thousand Oaks, CA: Corwin Press.

U.S. Department of Education (DOE). (1998). *Early Warning, Timely Response: A Guide to Safe Schools.* Washington, DC: Author.

U.S. Department of Health & Human Services (DHHS). (2003). *Bullying Is Not a Fact of Life.* Washington, DC: Author.

U.S. Secret Service (Secret Service) and U.S. Department of Education (DOE). (2002a). *The Final Report and Findings of the Safe School Initiative: Implications for the Prevention of School Attacks in the United States.* Washington, DC: Secret Service and DOE.

U.S. Secret Service (Secret Service) and U.S. Department of Education (DOE). (2002b). *Threat Assessment in Schools: A Guide to Managing Threatening Situations and to Creating Safe School Climates.* Washington, DC: Secret Service and DOE.

Van Dyke, J. M., & Sakurai, M. M. (2006). *Checklists for Searches and Seizures in Public Schools.* Eagan, MN: Thomson/West Publisher.

Index

115

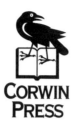

CORWIN PRESS

The Corwin Press logo—a raven striding across an open book—represents the union of courage and learning. Corwin Press is committed to improving education for all learners by publishing books and other professional development resources for those serving the field of PreK–12 education. By providing practical, hands-on materials, Corwin Press continues to carry out the promise of its motto: **"Helping Educators Do Their Work Better."**

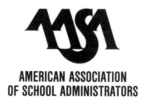

AMERICAN ASSOCIATION OF SCHOOL ADMINISTRATORS

The American Association of School Administrators, founded in 1865, is the professional organization for more than 13,000 educational leaders across the United States. AASA's mission is to support and develop effective school system leaders who are dedicated to the highest quality public education for all children. For more information, visit www.aasa.org.